25 MEDICAL TESTS
YOUR DOCTOR SHOULD TELL YOU ABOUT...
AND 15 YOU CAN DO YOURSELF

25 MEDICAL TESTS

YOUR DOCTOR SHOULD TELL YOU ABOUT...

AND 15 YOU CAN DO YOURSELF

Deborah Mitchell

A Lynn Sonberg Book

St. Martin's Paperbacks

Notice: This book is intended as a reference volume only, not as a medical manual. The information given here is designed to help you make informed decisions about your health. It is not intended as a substitute for any treatment that may have been prescribed by your doctor. If you suspect that you have a medical problem, we urge you to seek competent medical help.

Mention of specific companies, organizations, or authorities in this book does not imply endorsement by the author or publisher, nor does mention of specific companies, organizations, or authorities imply that they endorse this book, its author or the publisher.

Internet addresses given in this book were accurate at the time it went to press.

25 MEDICAL TESTS YOUR DOCTOR SHOULD TELL YOU ABOUT . . . AND 15 YOU CAN DO YOURSELF

Copyright © 2010 by Lynn Sonberg Book Associates.

Cover photograph of stethoscope by Getty Images/Jeffrey Hamilton.

All rights reserved.

For information address St. Martin's Press, 175 Fifth Avenue, New York, NY 10010.

EAN: 978-0-312-37314-6

Printed in the United States of America

St. Martin's Paperbacks edition / January 2010

St. Martin's Paperbacks are published by St. Martin's Press, 175 Fifth Avenue, New York, NY 10010.

10 9 8 7 6 5 4 3 2 1

TABLE OF CONTENTS

CHAPTER 1

WHAT YOU NEED TO KNOW ABOUT MEDICAL TESTS

It's a common occurrence: you walk into your doctor's office with a complaint and you walk out with one or more orders for tests: blood work, X-rays, scans—you name it. Perhaps you are given a piece of paper with a list of instructions: don't eat or drink anything for a specific number of hours before the test, be sure to drink a specific formula before the test, don't wear jewelry or powder, and so on.

Or maybe you are admitted into a hospital where you are poked, prodded, and then wheeled to different areas of the facility for various tests. In either case, your mind is racing with questions: Why do I need this test? What will the results tell me about my condition? How is the test done? Is it going to be painful? How do I prepare for it? Are there any side effects or precautions I need to consider?

Okay, now let's assume that the results of your tests have come in, and they should be shared with you. When they are, you may find yourself puzzled or confused by the explanation offered by the doctor or other health-care professional, and perhaps you are too embarrassed to ask questions or for clarification. You're not alone: many health-care consumers feel the same way.

But your health and that of your family is serious business, and you need and deserve to know about the tests you take and what they mean. That's why the goal of this book is to answer questions you and other health-care consumers have about some of the most common tests prescribed by health-care practitioners that are used to screen for or diagnose the more common diseases and conditions. In addition, we also introduce you to a rapidly growing segment of the health-care arena—self-testing, or home medical test kits. These are tests you can typically do at home, either by purchasing a test kit from your neighborhood pharmacy or from a company online. We have dedicated an entire chapter to this topic.

HOW DID WE CHOOSE THE TESTS IN THIS BOOK?

You may be wondering, of the hundreds of diagnostic and screening tests that are available, how and why did we choose the ones that are in this book? We used several criteria, including how often a test is ordered, the prevalence of the condition(s) for which it is used, the number of conditions it can diagnose or screen for, and its reliability. For example, the complete blood count (CBC) is one of the most ordered tests because it is often part of a routine checkup or screening, can be used as a follow-up procedure to monitor certain conditions or treatments, and is frequently part of an evaluation done to check on a patient's symptoms. A CBC is helpful in the diagnosis and screening of dozens of medical conditions, many of which are among the more common health problems people face, ranging from anemia to coronary heart disease to kidney infections.

Whether the test you need is done by a medical professional or by you at home, this book provides the most up-to-date information about these procedures so you can feel more confident when discussing them with your doctor or gathering health information for your own purposes. The information in this book can help you know which questions to ask your doctor, nurse, pharmacist, or other medical professional, and hopefully eliminate much of the mystery and any anxiety you may have about the tests.

In addition to explaining the nuts and bolts of several dozen tests, this book also has a section with entries on the more common medical conditions that the tests are used to identify or diagnose.

Overall, if you want to have more control over your health-care decisions, then this book is for you.

WHAT ARE MEDICAL TESTS?

Medical tests are a type of medical procedure that are prescribed for a variety of reasons, including diagnosing a specific disease or type of related condition, screening for disease, evaluating the severity of a disease, and monitoring the response to treatment. Frequently doctors will also order tests as a preventive measure as part of a routine examination to make sure everything is all right.

Tests can be performed to accomplish more than one purpose; for example, a blood test may reveal the presence of an infection, and it can also show whether a treatment is effective. Similarly, various types of scans may both identify an abnormality and also help your doctor monitor the efficacy of any therapy.

Types of Medical Tests

Depending on the source, medical tests can be classified into many different categories. We have chosen seven: analysis of body fluids, imaging, endoscopy, measurement of body functions, biopsy, genetic material analysis, and screening. Sometimes a test seems to qualify for more than one category; for example, endoscopy of the stomach lets clinicians examine the inside of the stomach and also capture a biopsy sample. Here is a brief explanation of the different types of medical tests:

Analysis of body fluids: Tests in this category involve the collection and analysis of blood, urine, cerebrospinal fluid (the fluid that surrounds the brain and spinal cord), saliva, sperm, vaginal fluids, digestive juices, and fluids that may collect in the stomach or near the lungs as a result of disease. A complete blood count (CBC) is probably the most commonly recognized test in this group.

Imaging: Regular X-rays are the most common type of imaging tests, but many other more sophisticated tests are often prescribed, including ultrasound, nuclear (radioisotope) scans, magnetic resonance imaging (MRI), positron-emission tomography (PET) scans, and computed tomography (CT) scans. These tests are designed to provide clinicians with images of the inside of the body.

Endoscopy: These tests utilize a special tube that usually has a camera and light at the tip. The tube is inserted into the body, usually through an existing body opening, and images of organs or cavities (spaces) are then viewed on a monitor by a clinician. Most endoscopes are flexible, although a few types are rigid. Some endoscopic procedures require tools be passed through the endoscope to remove tissue samples (biopsy).

Measurement of body functions: How is your heart functioning? How about your kidneys? There are a wide range of tests that record and analyze the activity of various body organs. An electrocardiogram (EKG), for example, measures the electrical activity of the heart, while an electroencephalogram (EEG) records the electrical activity of the brain.

Biopsy: A biopsy involves removing tissue samples from inside or outside the body and then examining them under a microscope. Tissues that are examined most often include skin, breast, liver, bone, kidney, and lung.

Genetic material analysis: Tests in this category involve evaluating cells from blood, skin, or bone marrow to see if there are any abnormalities in the genes, chromosomes, or both. Genetic testing is typically done in children and young adults to determine if they have a disease or are at risk of a disease, while adults may choose genetic testing to identify the likelihood of their children being born with or developing certain diseases.

Screening: Tests in this category are used to detect disease and other medical conditions in people who have no symptoms, and so it is easy to see why they often can be found in more than one category. Mammography, for example, is used for breast cancer screening, but is also considered an imaging test. Other types of screening tests include those that evaluate hearing and vision. Screening tests are designed to be sensitive (have the ability to detect many problems) but not specific (cannot identify the actual disease). That's why if the results of a screening test are positive, your doctor will schedule additional, more specific testing to identify the disease.

MEDICAL TESTS AND DEFENSIVE MEDICINE

Because they fear they will miss a diagnosis and expose themselves to malpractice lawsuits, many doctors are ordering expensive and unnecessary medical tests. This practice, known as defensive medicine, is estimated to cost more than $100 billion per year. One recent study shows that the next time you go into your doctor's office, you have a 43 percent chance of being ordered an unnecessary test. In many cases, patients end up paying for these tests because insurance companies are refusing to pick up the costs and/or because of increasingly rising copayment requirements.

What can you do? To protect yourself against undergoing costly, unneeded medical tests, ask yourself, your doctor, and a second physician (if you are not satisfied with the information you've gathered thus far) these questions before you agree to a test:

- Why is this test needed? Some doctors, for example, are known to order a computed tomography (CT) or magnetic resonance imaging (MRI) scan for every patient who complains of a headache. Yet brain tumors are rarely found in people who have headaches, so these tests are rarely necessary.

- Will the test results give the doctor information that will help him or her make

decisive treatment decisions? Or will another test—or no test at all—provide enough
information?

• How much does this test cost? Remember,
you may end up paying for the test.

• What risks do I expose myself to if I do not
have this test?

• What alternative tests are available that will
provide the same or similar information?
Often a less expensive and/or less invasive
test can provide the doctor the information
he or she needs.

HOW RELIABLE ARE MEDICAL TEST RESULTS?

As we noted previously, one of the criteria for the
tests chosen to be included in this book was reliability. Nothing is perfect, and that holds true for the
reliability of diagnostic and screening tests, the results of which can vary widely depending on various
factors. However, we selected tests that have been
shown to be as accurate, precise, sensitive, and specific as possible when done correctly. In many of the
entries, we have noted circumstances that may make
a particular test less reliable. For example, obesity
can make the results of an abdominal ultrasound
less accurate, and smoking cigarettes before an il-

licit drug test may compromise the reliability of this test. Now let's look at some of the factors that can impact the reliability of medical tests.

Four indicators are usually used to determine the reliability of clinical lab tests. Accuracy and precision both indicate how well the test method performs day to day in a laboratory. Sensitivity and specificity involve how well the test is able to distinguish whether a disease is present or absent in the person tested. Laboratory tests are designed to be as precise, accurate, sensitive, and specific as possible.

Let's consider **precision**. A test is said to be precise when it can be repeated many times on the same sample and give similar results each time. That means the amount of random variation among the results is small and the test is said to have good "repeatability."

A test method's **accuracy** is determined by how close the test value is to the absolute "true" value of the substance being measured. Results from every test that is done are compared to established control specimens that have undergone many evaluations and compared to the gold standard for that test.

We would all like to have tests that are 100 percent accurate and 100 percent precise, but in reality small discrepancies can occur. That's because there are some variations between laboratories and their methods, instrumentation, and level of staff training. This is one reason why if you have a test repeated for any reason, your doctor will want to use the same laboratory, to avoid introducing any variation in precision and accuracy.

The two critical components that determine a test's accuracy are sensitivity and specificity. **Sensitivity** is the probability that a test is positive, assuming that the person being tested has the disease. Therefore, a certain test may have proven to be 95 percent sensitive. If 100 people are known to have a certain disease, the test that identifies that disease will do so correctly for 95 of the 100 people tested. The other five people tested will not show the expected result for the test. For that 5 percent, the test result of "normal" will actually be an incorrect, *false-negative* result. That means those five people will believe they are disease free when in fact they are not. The more sensitive a test is, the fewer false-negative results it will produce. That's why clinicians want the most sensitive diagnostic tests possible. In many cases, if a person gets a test result that the doctor suspects may be a false-negative result, he or she may order another—often different—test to verify the first results.

Specificity is the ability of a test to correctly eliminate people who do not have a certain disease or condition. For example, a certain test may have proven to be 93 percent specific. If 100 healthy individuals are given the test, only 93 of the 100 will be found "normal" or get negative results (be disease free). The remaining seven people (who do not have the disease) will get positive test results. For these seven people (7%), their "abnormal" findings are *false-positive* results.

Obviously, getting a false-positive test result is a

problem, because no one wants to be treated for a disease that he or she does not have. Therefore, people who get a positive test result should contact their doctor to discuss the possibility that their results are a false-positive if they suspect the results may be in error, and ask what other testing they should have done to verify the results.

ONE LAST NOTE: THINK AHEAD

A question people need to ask themselves before undergoing a medical test is, What will I do with the information? When you and your doctor discuss your medical condition and any tests he or she may order, you should also discuss the treatment options you will have, depending on the results of the test(s). If, for example, your doctor orders a complete blood count because you may have anemia, you should know what treatment strategies are available to you. If you do not want to follow any of the doctor's treatment recommendations, even if you are told you have anemia, then you may want to think twice about having the test, or just have the test for your own information or until you change your mind about treatment.

In some cases, treatment options may include surgical procedures or additional testing. If you are undergoing a bronchoscopy and there is a possibility that you have lung cancer, you may want to think about researching surgeons in your area. If you are undergoing an amniocentesis because there is a possibility you are carrying a child with a genetic disorder, you should have a list of genetic counselors at your disposal so you can discuss your options with a knowledgeable individual.

The bottom line is that you should think carefully about any medical test you take: why and if you need it, how to prepare for it, what the risks are, and what you will do with the results. This book will help you with these questions.

CHAPTER 2

25 COMMON MEDICAL TESTS

ABDOMINAL ULTRASOUND
Why Do I Need This Test?

An abdominal ultrasound is an imaging test that uses high-frequency sound waves (rather than the ionizing radiation used in X-rays) to produce pictures of the organs and other structures in the upper abdomen. The test is used to evaluate the abdominal aorta and other blood vessels in the abdomen, kidneys, liver, gallbladder, pancreas, and spleen. An abdominal ultrasound can help diagnose various problems, including abdominal pain, an enlarged abdomen, kidney stones, stones in the gallbladder, abnormal liver function, urinary blockage, trauma to the abdomen, an obvious or suspected abdominal mass, and an abdominal aortic aneurysm (symptoms include belly or chest pain, pulsating sensation in the abdomen). Sometimes an abdominal ultrasound is used to help clinicians perform needle biopsies, in which needles are used to take tissue samples from any of the organs mentioned above.

In some cases, doctors also do a Doppler ultrasound study as part of an abdominal ultrasound examination. Doppler ultrasound is a special technique that evaluates how blood flows through a blood vessel, including the major arteries and veins in the abdomen, legs, neck, and arms.

What Will the Results Tell Me?

Your clinician will be able to observe and evaluate the presence of blood clots or other blockages to blood flow, presence of tumors or congenital abnormalities, and narrowing of blood vessels. Possible conditions an abdominal ultrasound can reveal include abdominal aortic aneurysm, cholecystitis (inflammation of the gallbladder caused by stones in that organ), gallstones, hydronephrosis (swollen or distended kidney), kidney stones, splenomegaly (enlarged spleen), or pancreatitis.

Abdominal ultrasound results may not be as accurate in patients who are very overweight, because the sound waves cannot pass as easily through large amounts of fatty tissue.

How Do I Prepare for the Test?

Depending on which organs your doctor needs to view, you may be asked to do the following:

• To study your liver, gallbladder, spleen, or pancreas, you may be asked to eat a fat-free meal the evening before the test and to refrain from eating anything for 8–12 hours before the test. It is important to avoid any accumulation of gas in the intestines because it can prevent visualization of the pancreas. Also, fasting allows the gallbladder to be seen because it contracts after eating and thus usually cannot be seen when the stomach is full.

• To study your kidneys, you may be asked to drink 4–6 glasses of water about an hour before the test and to avoid eating for 8–12 hours before the test to avoid any accumulation of gas in the intestinal tract.

• To view the aorta, you will need to avoid eating for 8–12 hours before the test.

Tell your doctor if you have undergone any upper gastrointestinal tests or a barium enema within two days of your scheduled test. Any barium that remains in the intestinal tract can prevent an accurate ultrasound reading.

You will need to remove all clothing and jewelry in the area to be examined and will be asked to wear a gown during the test.

What Happens During the Test?

During the ultrasound test, you will likely lie faceup on an examination table that can be moved or tilted. An ultrasound technologist (sonographer) will apply a clear gel to the area to be examined. The gel allows the transducer to make good contact with the body. A transducer is a small handheld device that the technologist presses against the skin and moves back and forth over the area as it transmits high-frequency sound waves into the body. You may be asked to change position during the test or to hold your breath for a few seconds.

As the sound waves bounce off the structures inside the body, the microphone in the transducer records the returning echoes from the tissues and displays them in real time on a monitor. Some of the images are captured as still photos. The entire ultrasound testing procedure takes about 30 minutes. An abdominal ultrasound is usually painless unless you have some tenderness in your abdominal area, in which case you may experience some mild and temporary discomfort.

If Doppler ultrasound is also part of the study, a computer will collect and process the sounds and images of the blood as it flows through the blood vessels and measure the direction and speed of the blood cells as they flow.

What Happens After the Test?

Once the technologist has completed the test, he or she will wipe the gel off your body. Because the test is conducted in real time, you may get your results immediately from a radiologist (a physician who specializes in interpreting radiology tests), or the radiologist may send the results to your physician, who will share the results with you. There are no adverse effects from an abdominal ultrasound, and you may return to your regular activities immediately after the test.

What Are the Risks?
There are no risks associated with an abdominal ultrasound.

AMNIOCENTESIS
Why Do I Need This Test?
An amniocentesis is a prenatal diagnostic test that is usually performed during weeks 15–18 of pregnancy, although it can be performed as early as 11 weeks. It is the most commonly prescribed invasive test during pregnancy in the United States. An amniocentesis is recommended for women older than 35, since they have greater risk of giving birth to a child with chromosomal defects, including Down syndrome, trisomy 13, and Turner syndrome. However, a woman of any age can request an amniocentesis, especially if there is a history of genetic disorders in her family. An amniocentesis can also detect genetic disorders, including cystic fibrosis, and neural tube defects, the most common of which is spina bifida.

You may also use this test if you need to determine paternity. Amniocentesis allows collection of DNA from the fetus, which can be compared to DNA from the potential father.

What Will the Results Tell Me?

Depending on the types of analyses you and your doctor have requested, you can learn the gender of your infant, the presence of a number of abnormalities, and paternity. For example, an elevated alpha-fetoprotein (AFP) level may indicate a defect in brain and spinal-cord development, such as spina bifida, while a low AFP level may indicate Down syndrome. Any abnormal levels of AFP are an indication that your doctor should look for chromosomal abnormalities and birth defects. An amniocentesis is more than 99 percent accurate in predicting chromosomal disorders and in determining paternity.

Physicians are able to test for lung maturity, which can help your doctor make a decision regarding the timing of delivery if premature labor is a possibility, or for women who have diabetes or other medical conditions that require early delivery. Pregnant women who have fever without an obvious infection may also undergo amniocentesis to determine if the fever is from an intrauterine infection.

Amniocentesis can also help identify specific genetic conditions, such as Tay-Sachs disease, cystic fibrosis, sickle-cell anemia, and other inherited disorders. Such testing is not performed routinely, but is available upon request. Amniocentesis cannot detect defects such as hernia, cleft lip, or extra fingers or toes. Ultrasound is the only test that can detect these defects.

How Do I Prepare for the Test?

You will be asked to sign a consent form before the procedure is done. Although there are no food or liquid restrictions before taking the test, a full bladder is necessary for the ultrasound.

What Happens During the Test?

The test is performed by inserting a hollow needle through the abdominal wall into the uterus and withdrawing a small amount of amniotic fluid (usually about 1 cc per week of gestation) from the sac that surrounds the fetus. The test is usually guided by ultrasound to make sure the doctor knows where he or she should insert the needle. If the doctor uses an anesthetic, you will feel a sharp stinging sensation when the anesthetic needle is inserted. When the hollow needle enters the amniotic sac, you may feel a sharp pain that lasts only a few seconds. Some women experience a sensation of pressure in the lower abdomen when the doctor withdraws the fluid.

What Happens After the Test?

Some women have mild, temporary cramping after the procedure, which can be relieved with an over-the-counter pain reliever. You can return to your normal schedule immediately after the amniocentesis unless you feel unwell.

Results usually take up to several weeks, depending on the analyses requested.

What Are the Risks?

The risk of miscarriage is approximately 1 in 1,600 pregnancies, according to a recent study (2006) conducted by experts at Mount Sinai School of Medicine. This study refutes the older rate of 0.5 percent, or 1 in 200 pregnancies. There is also a slight risk of infection from the procedure by introducing bacteria through the needle site. Leaking of amniotic fluid also can occur, although this risk is rare.

Another rare risk is Rh incompatibility. If the amniocentesis causes an exchange of blood between the fetus and the mother, which can occur if the placenta is accidentally pricked during the test, it can trigger an Rh response, causing the mother's immune system to attack the fetus.

BARIUM ENEMA
Why Do I Need This Test?

A barium enema is an X-ray test that allows clinicians to examine the lower digestive tract (colon and rectum). Because the colon and rectum cannot be seen on X-rays, barium is used to temporarily coat the inner surfaces. A barium enema may help diagnose cancers and small sacs called diverticula that can form in the intestinal walls.

There are two types of barium enemas. A single-contrast study involves filling the colon with barium, which can reveal large abnormalities. In a double-contrast study, the colon is filled with barium and then most of it is drained out, leaving a coating of barium on the colon walls. The colon is then filled with air, which provides a more detailed view of the inner surface of the colon.

Your doctor may order a barium enema to:

• Screen for colon polyps or colon cancer

• Identify inflammation of the intestinal wall, which is characteristic of inflammatory bowel diseases (ulcerative colitis, Crohn's disease)

• Detect structural problems, such as sacs (diverticula) in the intestinal wall

• Help explain changed bowel habits, anemia, or unexplained weight loss

What Will the Results Tell Me?

You should get your results within a day or two. If the results of a single-contrast study are not clear or there is a strong suspicion of cancer, your doctor may order a double-contrast study.

Abnormal findings may indicate:

• Narrowing or obstruction in the bowel

• Inflammation of the lining of the colon (colitis)

• Sacs in the colon wall (diverticulosis)

- An area of the colon that did not fill with barium, suggesting a blockage

- Twisted loop of bowel

- Intussusception (rare but serious obstruction of the bowel) in a child. A barium enema may be used to treat the bowel and return it to normal position.

How Do I Prepare for the Test?

Tell your doctor if you might be or are pregnant. If you need to take insulin for diabetes, discuss this with your doctor before the test.

It is important that your colon be completely empty before the barium enema. The day before the test you will likely be told to consume liquids only (including plain gelatin, juices, and broth—but no dairy) and to drink a large amount of clear liquids between meals. You will need to take a laxative that will help empty your colon. On the day of the barium enema, do not eat any breakfast.

What Happens During the Test?

You will need to disrobe and wear a hospital gown. While you lie on your side on a table in the radiology department, a nurse will push a small lubricated tube an inch or two into your rectum. The barium liquid enters your intestinal tract through the tube. You will feel pressure, like you need to have a bowel movement, but the procedure is not painful.

As soon as the enema begins, a large camera that is positioned over your abdomen begins to take an X-ray video. A doctor watches the video and may ask you to hold your breath for a few seconds when he or she wants to save an image. You also may be asked to turn to different positions, and the table may be tilted so pictures can be taken from different directions. If a double-contrast study is being done, the barium will be drained out and your colon will be filled with air. You may experience some cramping and gas pains.

When the test is done, the enema tube is removed and you will be allowed to go to the toilet to eliminate as much of the barium as you can. One or two additional X-ray images may be taken after you have gotten rid of the barium.

A single-contrast study usually takes 30–45 minutes, although the barium is inside only about 15 minutes. A double-contrast study may take up to 60 minutes.

What Happens After the Test?

You may feel tired after the test and your anal area may be sore for a day or two. A local anesthetic ointment can ease any discomfort. Drink plenty of fluids to replace those you lost during the test. Your bowel movements may look white or pink for several days after the test.

What Are the Risks?

No significant risks are associated with a barium enema. You will be exposed to radiation during the test, equaling more than a simple chest X-ray but still a small amount. In rare cases side effects occur. Call your doctor immediately if you have rectal bleeding, severe abdominal pain, fever, or do not have a bowel movement within two days after the test.

BONE DENSITY TEST
Why Do I Need This Test?

A bone mineral density (BMD) test, also called bone densitometry, is done to identify people who have osteoporosis or who are at risk of osteoporosis. It uses special X-rays to measure how many grams of calcium and other bone minerals are found in the bone of the area tested. These tests are sometimes confused with bone scans, which are used to detect fractures, cancer, infections, and bone abnormalities.

The National Osteoporosis Foundation recommends that people have a bone density test if they meet the following conditions:

• You are a woman older than age 65

• You are postmenopausal, younger than 65, and have at least one risk factor for osteoporosis, including having a fractured bone

• You have X-ray evidence of a spinal fracture or bone loss

• You experienced early menopause

- You are taking drugs that can cause osteo-porosis, such as prednisone

- You are a man 50 to 70 who has one or more risk factors for osteoporosis

- You are a man age 70 or older, even without risk factors

- You have hyperparathyroidism or hyperthy-roidism

Research has not determined how often people should undergo bone density screenings or when screening can stop. However, experts generally agree that two or more years between tests are needed to accurately measure a change in bone density. You should check with your physician to determine the best screening interval for you based on your medical history and current health status.

A bone density test can be done two ways: periph-erally or centrally. A peripheral device usually tests for bone density in the heel while a central device tests the spine and hips. The latter is called a dual-energy X-ray absorptiometry (DEXA) scan. It is more accurate than a peripheral scan, but it is also more expensive. If you have a positive test result on a pe-ripheral test, your doctor will likely recommend you get a DEXA.

What Will the Results Tell Me?

Results of the test will tell you your risk for osteoporosis. If you have the test done using a peripheral device, you can usually get the results immediately. If, however, you have a DEXA, results are typically available within a few days.

Results will include two scores: T-score and Z-score. The T-score is a measure of your bone density compared with the average values in young adults of the same sex and race. The Z-score shows you how your bone density compares with that of people your own sex, age, and race. A positive T-score means your bones are stronger than the average young adult, and a negative score means they are weaker. Up to −1.0 is considered normal. If your T-score is between −1.0 and −2.5, you have osteopenia. If it is below −2.5, you have osteoporosis.

If you have osteopenia (bone mineral density that is lower than normal but not yet classified as osteoporosis) or osteoporosis, you can begin treatment and lifestyle changes that can help slow progression of the disease. Generally, the lower your bone density, the greater your risk of experiencing a fracture. Bone density that is measured at the hip and spine is considered to be the best predictor of hip and spine fracture. This is critical because hip fractures are very disabling, and spine fractures are common and painful. However, wrist fractures are also very common in people who have osteopenia or osteoporosis.

This test is also helpful for monitoring progress if you are taking bone-building medications.

How Do I Prepare for the Test?

Tell your doctor if you are pregnant, because X-rays used during pregnancy can result in birth defects, even though the radiation emitted during DEXA is about one-tenth that given during a regular chest X-ray.

If you have had oral contrast or nuclear medicine tests done recently, tell your doctor before you undergo DEXA because these tests can interfere with a bone density test.

What Happens During the Test?

You will lie on a padded platform or table for a few minutes while an imager passes over your body. The instrument does not touch your body, but it does emit radiation. The test usually takes 5–10 minutes to complete.

What Happens After the Test?

You can resume your regular activities immediately after the test.

What are the Risks?

Bone density testing has no risks. Although the test can confirm that you have low bone density, it cannot tell you why. Your doctor will need to do a complete medical evaluation to determine the cause.

BRONCHOSCOPY
Why Do I Need This Test?

A bronchoscopy is a test that allows your doctor to view your airway, including your throat, larynx, trachea, and lower airways, through a thin instrument called a bronchoscope. It may be used to diagnose problems with the airway or to treat conditions such as a growth in the airway. Bronchoscopy is typically performed when a doctor suspects lung disease and needs to inspect the airways or take a sample to confirm it. For example, bronchoscopy can be used to:

- Identify the cause of problems in your airway, such as bleeding, chronic cough, or breathing problems

- Take tissue samples when other tests, such as X-rays, indicate problems in the lungs

- Diagnose lung diseases by collecting sputum or tissue samples

- Remove objects that are blocking the airway

- Diagnose lung cancer

- Evaluate and treat growth in the airway

- Control bleeding in the airway

- Treat cancer of the airway

What Will the Results Tell Me?

The doctor may discuss the results with you immediately after the test is done. If a biopsy was taken, the results will take about 2–4 days. If the results are normal, this means that the airway leading to your lungs and the breathing tubes in your lungs appear normal, with no thick secretions, growths, or objects.

Abnormal results can mean there is an abnormality in the bronchial wall, enlarged tubular vessels, enlarged lymph nodes or glands, hemorrhaging, infection (from bacteria, viruses, fungi, or parasites), irregular bronchial branching, lung cancer, narrowing of the trachea, inflammation, tumor, or ulceration.

How Do I Prepare for the Test?

You will be asked to sign a consent form before the test. Tell your doctor about any medications, allergies to medications, bleeding problems, or if you are pregnant before you take the test. Do not drink or eat for at least 8–10 hours before the test.

Immediately before the test you should remove any dentures, eyeglasses, contact lenses, hearing aids, wigs, makeup, and jewelry. Also empty your bladder. You will be asked to remove all or most of your clothes and put on a gown.

What Happens During the Test?

Before the test begins, you may be given a chest X-ray. The test is done by a pulmonologist and an assistant. Throughout the procedure your blood pressure, oxygen level, and heart rate will be monitored.

There are two types of bronchoscopy, flexible and rigid. The procedures are slightly different for each one.

Flexible bronchoscopy. You will be given medication to dry up the secretions in your mouth and airway. A bronchoscopy can be done with you either lying down on a table, reclining in a chair, or sitting upright. You will be given a sedative, and an intravenous (IV) line may be placed in your arm. Throughout the procedure you will be awake but drowsy. The doctor will spray a local anesthetic into your nose and mouth, which will numb your throat and help reduce your gag reflex. If the bronchoscope is inserted through your nose, the doctor may put an anesthetic ointment in your nose as well.

The doctor will gently and slowly insert the bronchoscope through your mouth or nose and toward your vocal cords. You may be asked to take a deep breath to help the scope pass your vocal cords. A fluoroscope (a type of X-ray machine) may be brought above you to take X-ray images, which will help the doctor as he or she collects samples from your lung. The bronchoscope is then moved down to your bronchi to examine the lower airways. You may feel some pressure in your airway as the bronchoscope is moved during the test.

If your doctor is gathering sputum or tissue samples for biopsy, he or she may use a tiny device through the scope to gather them. Small biopsy forceps may be used to remove lung tissue samples.

Rigid bronchoscopy. This test is usually done under general anesthesia and while you lie on your back on a table. You will be given a sedative and an intravenous (IV) line will be placed in your arm. The doctor will also place an endotracheal tube in your windpipe, which is hooked up to a machine that will help you breathe during the procedure. You will feel nothing during the procedure, due to the anesthesia.

Once you are asleep, the doctor will position your head with your neck extended and then gently and slowly insert the bronchoscope through your mouth and into your throat. If your doctor is collecting tissue or sputum samples, a tiny device will be passed through the scope.

What Happens After the Test?

You will be in recovery for 2–3 hours after the test. It is recommended that you have someone drive you home. Until you can swallow without choking, you should spit out any saliva and not eat or drink anything (usually about 2 hours). When you do resume your normal diet, start by taking small sips of water. If you smoke, do not start for at least 24 hours after the test.

You may feel tired for a day or two and have some muscle aches after the procedure. If you were given a local anesthetic, you may have a bitter taste in your mouth for a day or so. You may also experience a sore throat and hoarseness for a few days. If the doctor took a biopsy sample, it is normal to spit up a small amount of blood after the test.

What Are the Risks?

Bronchoscopy is usually a safe procedure. Complications are rare, and may include:

- Irregular heart rhythms

- Infection, such as pneumonia

- Chronic hoarseness

- Bronchial tube spasms, which can make breathing difficult

If your doctor took a biopsy during the test, complications that may occur include:

- Bleeding caused by the use of biopsy forceps

- Infection

- A very small chance of death

- Pneumothorax (partial collapse of the lung) caused by air getting into the pleural space from a tear in the lung from the biopsy forceps

Call your doctor immediately if you cough up more than 2 tablespoons of blood, have trouble breathing, or if you have a fever greater than 100°F for more than 24 hours. A mild fever (lower than 100°F) is common right after the procedure.

CARDIAC CATHETERIZATION WITH CORONARY ANGIOGRAM

Why Do I Need This Test?

Cardiac catheterization with coronary angiogram takes images of the blood vessels in the heart and uses a special dye to locate any problems in the coronary arteries. The test is usually performed by a cardiologist or a radiologist and allows clinicians to evaluate the health status of the heart and identify any narrowing or obstructions of the blood vessels.

What Will the Results Tell Me?

The results can show if you have any blocked coronary arteries, how many are affected and how severe the problem is, and the best way to treat them. In some cases, the blockages can be removed immediately with a procedure called coronary angioplasty, in which a tiny inflatable balloon is used to reopen the blood vessel.

How Do I Prepare for This Test?

You may be asked to not eat anything for 6–8 hours before the test to reduce the risk that you may become nauseated and vomit during the procedure. Before the test, tell your doctor if you take nonsteroidal anti-inflammatory drugs (NSAIDs) or any other medications that affect blood clotting, or if you take insulin shots or antidiabetes drugs. You should also tell your doctor if you have ever had an allergic reaction to local anesthetics or contrast dyes, or if you are pregnant.

What Happens During the Test?

You will lie on your back on a table and a medical technician will place an intravenous (IV) line in your arm so you can be given a sedative to help you relax. You will also be connected to a heart monitor. The cardiologist will inject a local anesthetic into your skin where the catheter (a thin, hollow plastic tube) will be inserted. This is typically in the groin area.

When your skin is numb, the doctor will insert the catheter into a large artery and move it along until it reaches your aorta. He or she will do this using live images displayed on a monitor as a guide. When the tip of the catheter reaches one of your coronary arteries, the doctor will inject contrast dye through the catheter. The dye will make it possible for the doctor to see if the artery is blocked or narrowed. This procedure is repeated for the other coronary arteries as well.

During the test, X-ray images will be taken to monitor the dye as it moves through the arteries. In some cases, a contrast dye may be injected into the left ventricle of the heart to show how hard your heart is pumping. After the catheter is withdrawn, the doctor will use a stitch to prevent bleeding from the entry site. The entire test takes 1 hour or longer.

What Happens After the Test?

After the test, you should lie flat for several hours. You will feel sleepy from the sedatives, and you should not drive or drink alcohol for at least 24 hours after the catheterization.

What Are the Risks?

This test has several potential risks. The catheter may irritate the heart, which can cause the coronary artery to go into spasm and produce chest pain. Therefore, if you experience any chest discomfort or other pain during the test, tell the doctors and nurses immediately. In rare cases, the catheter can disturb heart rhythm. If this occurs, the doctor can immediately restore normal rhythm with medications and devices. Other rare risks may include infection, stroke, blood clots, heart attack, irregular heart rythms, and bleeding around the entry point.

Use of the contrast medium rarely impairs kidney function. When it does, it is usually temporary. Some people are allergic to the contrast dye and develop a rash, hives, or breathing difficulty. If this occurs, the health professionals on hand will have medications to treat allergic reactions. Another possible complication is the formation of a bruise called a hematoma where the catheter was inserted. This usually resolves on its own.

COLONOSCOPY

Why Do I Need This Test?

A colonoscopy is a test used to view the inside of the colon and rectum. The test can detect inflamed tissue, abnormal growths in the intestinal tract, and ulcers. The test can look for early signs of colorectal cancer and help your doctor diagnose unexplained changes in bowel habits, bleeding from the anus, weight loss, unexplained anemia, persistent diarrhea, and abdominal pain. Routine colonoscopy is recommended for people beginning at age 50, and earlier if you have a family history of colorectal cancer, a personal history of inflammatory bowel disease, or other risk factors.

What Will the Results Tell Me?

If your doctor finds no abnormalities, you can probably wait several years before you have a repeat colonoscopy. Abnormal results can mean the presence of diverticulosis, polyps, inflammatory bowel disease, or a tumor (cancer). If abnormal tissue or polyps were found and they could not be removed during the procedure, your doctor may recommend surgery.

How Do I Prepare for the Test?

Your doctor should provide you with written instructions on how to prepare for the test. Preparation involves a bowel prep, which means all solids must be eliminated from the gastrointestinal tract by following a clear liquid diet for 1–3 days before the procedure. You should not drink any liquids that contain red or purple dye. Acceptable liquids include plain coffee and tea, strained fruit juice, fat-free broth or bouillon, water, sports drinks, and gelatin. You may also need to take a laxative or an enema the night before the colonoscopy.

At least one week before the procedure, tell your doctor if you have any medical conditions and which medications, vitamins, or supplements you take regularly. If you have diabetes or take blood thinners, for example, your doctor may have different preparation instructions for you.

You should make arrangements for a ride home because you are not permitted to drive for 12 hours after a colonoscopy to allow the sedative to wear off.

What Happens During the Test?

Many people refuse to have a colonoscopy because they have heard that it is painful, yet it can be relatively painless when it is done by an experienced clinician. It is also customary to administer a mild sedative either alone or along with an opiate painkiller to help minimize any discomfort.

You will need to remove your clothing and put on a gown. During the test you will likely lie on your left side. Your doctor will insert a colonoscope into your rectum. The colonoscope has a light on the tip and a channel that allows the doctor to send air into your colon. This may cause some abdominal cramping and pressure.

The colonoscope also has a video camera on its tip, and it sends images back to a monitor so your doctor can get a good view of the interior of your colon. If the doctor needs to remove polyps, take a tissue sample, or inject solutions, he or she can do so through the colonoscope. Depending on whether your doctor finds anything that needs attention during the test, a colonoscopy usually takes about 20–60 minutes.

What Happens After the Test?

After the test is over, it takes about 1 hour to partially recover from the sedative and about 24 hours for the effects to completely wear off. You will feel bloated and experience flatulence for several hours after the test. You can reduce your discomfort by walking. You may see a small amount of blood in the first bowel movement after the test. This is not unusual. However, if bleeding persists, if you pass blood clots, experience abdominal pain, or have a fever of 100°F or higher, contact your doctor as soon as possible.

What Are the Risks?

Although rare, a perforation (tear or hole) of the colon wall can occur if an instrument punctures the intestine during the procedure. Small tears that are found early may be treated with bowel rest, antibiotics, and careful monitoring. A large tear requires surgery.

Bleeding occurs in about 1 out of every 1,000 colonoscopy procedures. In most cases the bleeding resolves on its own. If your doctor has removed a polyp, there is a 30–50 percent chance bleeding will occur from 2 to 7 days after the test. This type of bleeding may also resolve on its own, but severe bleeding may require treatment.

Post-polypectomy syndrome may occur if the colon wall is burned during polyp removal. Symptoms of this syndrome include fever, abdominal pain, and an elevated white blood cell count anywhere from 12–48 hours after the procedure. Risk of infection after a colonoscopy is very low.

COMPLETE BLOOD COUNT
Why Do I Need This Test?

A complete blood count (CBC) is one of the most common and well-recognized medical tests. This broad screening tool is actually a panel of tests that examines many different parts of the blood to look for a wide variety of conditions, from anemia to infections and a host of others that can be detected in the blood and its components.

A baseline complete blood count test is recommended for everyone so there is a record of your general health status. If the various blood cell populations are within normal limits, then you may not need another CBC until your health changes or your doctor orders one. Your doctor may order a CBC if you are experiencing fatigue, weakness, inflammation, or bleeding, or if you have an infection. It can also be used to look for leukemia, a low fluid state (dehydration), and to manage chemotherapy decisions.

What Will the Results Tell Me?

Results of a CBC can be very revealing. Significant increases in white blood count, for example, may confirm the presence of an infection and suggest that further testing be done to identify the cause. Declines in red blood cell count can indicate anemia, while a low or extremely high platelet count may confirm the cause of clotting or excessive bleeding and can be associated with leukemia or other bone marrow diseases.

When you get your lab report you will see several

columns of numbers. One will be the values from your blood test and another will contain a reference range. The reference range of numbers is the range of values of the median 95 percent of the healthy population considering age, sex, and the method used in the testing laboratory. Having numbers outside any of the reference ranges does not mean you are sick. Results of a CBC are only a tool and typically just one part of an examination or quest for a diagnosis. You should discuss your CBC results with your physician. For an idea of what the acronyms in the report mean and the reference ranges, refer to the box, "Components of a CBC."

How Do I Prepare for the Test?

There is no special preparation needed for this test. Since blood is usually withdrawn from the arm, it is helpful to wear a shirt or top that can allow easy access. Tell your doctor about any medications you take because they may affect the outcome of the test.

What Happens During the Test?

A complete blood count can be done in a doctor's office, laboratory, hospital, clinic, or other appropriate location. A health-care professional usually draws the blood from a vein located on the inside of the arm near the elbow. First the skin surface is cleaned with an alcohol pad and an elastic band is placed around the upper arm, which causes the veins to swell with blood. A needle is inserted into a vein and blood is withdrawn by a syringe or a connection into a special vacuumed vial. One to two teaspoons of blood is the typical sample size. Once the blood has been withdrawn, the elastic band is removed and the collection site is covered with a bandage to stop any bleeding.

What Happens After the Test?

You should be able to return to your normal routine immediately after the test. However, in some cases individuals feel slightly light-headed for a few minutes after blood is drawn.

What Are the Risks?

A complete blood test is considered a very safe procedure. However, there are some problems that may occur when blood is drawn, such as feeling faint or light-headed, development of a hematoma (blood that accumulates under the skin, resulting in a lump or bruise), or pain associated with the health-care professional having to make several attempts at locating a vein.

Components of a CBC

• White blood cell (WBC) count: Count of the actual number of white blood cells per volume of blood. Both increases and decreases can be significant. Range: 4,300–10,800 cells/mcL (cells per) cubic millimeter

• White blood cell (WBC) differential: Looks at the types of white blood cells. Each of the five different types of white blood cells has its own function, although they all fight infection. The five types are neutrophils, lymphocytes, monocytes, eosinophils, and basophils.

- Red blood cell (RBC) count: Count of the actual number of red blood cells per blood volume. Range: 4.2–6.9 million/cells/mcL

- Red cell distribution width (RDW): A calculation of the variation in red blood cell size. In some types of anemia, such as pernicious anemia, the amount of variation in size of the red blood cells causes an increase in the RDW.

- Hemoglobin (Hgb): Amount of oxygen-carrying protein in the blood. Range: 13–18 gm/dL (grams per deciliter) for males; 12–16 gm/dL for females

- Hematocrit (HCT): Percentage of red blood cells in a given volume of whole blood. Range: 40–52% for males; 37–48% for females

- Platelet count: Number of platelets in a given volume of blood. The mean platelet volume (MPV) is the average size of your platelets. New platelets are larger than old ones, and an increased MPV occurs when more platelets are being manufactured. MPV indicates platelet production in your bone marrow. Range for platelet count: 150,000–400,000/platelets/microliter.

• Mean corpuscular volume (MCV): Measurement of the average size of your red blood cells. Red blood cells that are larger or smaller than average indicate various problems, such as vitamin B12 deficiency (larger than normal) or iron deficiency anemia (smaller). Range: 86–98 femtoliters

• Mean corpuscular hemoglobin (MCH): Calculation of the average amount of oxygen-carrying hemoglobin inside a red blood cell. Large red blood cells have a higher MCH than smaller ones. Range: 27–32 pg/cell (picograms per cell)

• Mean corpuscular hemoglobin concentration (MCHC): Calculation of the average concentration of hemoglobin inside red blood cells. High and low MCHC values can indicate various conditions; for example, iron deficiency anemia is characterized by low values while burn patients typically have high values. Range: 32–36% hemoglobin/cell

COMPREHENSIVE METABOLIC PANEL
Why Do I Need This Test?

A comprehensive metabolic panel (CMP) consists of 14 specific tests that are approved and recognized by Medicare and the majority of insurance companies, although individual labs may adjust the number of tests. Your doctor may order this panel to gather important information about the status of your liver, kidneys, electrolyte and acid/base balance, blood sugar, and blood proteins.

This panel is a broad-based screening tool that can check for conditions such as liver disease, diabetes, and kidney disease. Doctors routinely order a CMP as part of blood workup for a medical examination or yearly physical.

What Will the Results Tell Me?

The CMP measures the following substances: glucose, calcium, proteins (albumin, total protein), electrolytes (sodium, potassium, carbon dioxide, bicarbonate, chloride), kidney factors (blood urea nitrogen, creatinine), and liver factors (alkaline phosphatase, alanine aminotransferase, aspartate aminotransferase, bilirubin). (Also see "Glucose Testing" and "Liver Panel.") If any of the results are abnormal, your doctor may order follow-up tests to confirm or rule out a suspected diagnosis.

How Do I Prepare for the Test?

You should refrain from food and liquids (except water) for 10–12 hours before the test. If you routinely take medications, talk to your doctor about whether you should take them before the test.

What Happens During the Test?
A health-care professional usually draws the blood from a vein located on the inside of the arm near the elbow. First the skin surface is cleaned with an alcohol pad and an elastic band is placed around the upper arm, which causes the veins to swell with blood. A needle is inserted into a vein and blood is withdrawn by a syringe or a connection into a special vacuumed vial. One to two teaspoons of blood is the typical sample size. Once the blood has been withdrawn, the elastic band is removed and the collection site is covered with a bandage to stop any bleeding.

What Happens After the Test?
You should be able to return to your normal routine immediately after the test. However, in some cases individuals feel slightly light-headed for a few minutes after blood is drawn.

What Are the Risks?
A comprehensive metabolic panel is considered a very safe procedure. However, there are some problems that may occur when blood is drawn, such as feeling faint or light-headed, development of a hematoma (blood that accumulates under the skin, resulting in a lump or bruise), or pain associated with the health-care professional having to make several attempts at locating a vein.

ELECTROCARDIOGRAM
Why Do I Need This Test?

An electrocardiogram (EKG, sometimes referred to as ECG) is especially useful for diagnosing heart attack, heart failure, and abnormal heart rhythms. However, it can also provide information about other conditions associated with heart function. It is recommended that you have an EKG every one to three years after age 40 if you have heart disease; if you are at risk for developing heart disease because of diabetes, high blood pressure, or high cholesterol; or if you want to start a vigorous exercise regimen. Your doctor may recommend an EKG if you have signs and symptoms of a heart problem, including chest pain, heart palpitations, breathing problems, feelings of fatigue, and/or feelings of weakness. One may also be recommended if you have a history of heart disease in your family, especially if your mother, father, and/or siblings had the disease early in life.

An EKG can be used to monitor how well you are responding to heart medication or a medical device, such as a pacemaker. It is also usually ordered before major surgery as a screening tool.

What Will the Results Tell Me?

An EKG can detect many different heart problems. The recordings can help doctors diagnose a heart attack as it is happening or one that has occurred in the past. This is especially true if you have a past

EKG recording with which your current one can be compared.

An EKG can also show:

- Lack of blood flow to the heart

- Heart failure

- Arrhythmia (abnormal rhythm)

- Heart muscle that is abnormally thick

- Heart is abnormally large

- Birth defects in the heart

- Heart valve disease

- Pericarditis (inflammation of the sac around the heart)

How Do I Prepare for the Test?

There are no special preparations. If you have a hairy chest, a nurse may have to shave several patches so the stickers (leads or electrodes) can be stuck to your skin. Because some medications may affect the outcome of an EKG, tell your doctor about any drugs you are taking.

What Happens During the Test?

An EKG can be done in a doctor's office, clinic, or hospital. You will lie on your back with your shirt off, and stickers will be stuck to your chest in a row and then in one place on each arm and leg. The leads record electrical activity from your heart, and do not send any type of electrical current to your body. The results are printed out on a sheet of paper as the information is transmitted over the leads. You must remain still during the test, which takes three to four minutes, but you will not feel anything. If you experience any chest pain during the test, tell the person who is taking the EKG.

What Happens After the Test?

When the test is over, the nurse will remove the electrodes from your skin. You may experience a mild rash or redness where the leads were attached. This usually disappears quickly without treatment. You can return to your regular routine immediately after the test.

A doctor can interpret an EKG immediately after the test is done. However, if a technician does the EKG and no doctor is present, you may not get your results for several days until a cardiologist interprets them for you.

What Are the Risks?

There are no risks or pain associated with an EKG.

ELECTROMYOGRAPHY AND NERVE CONDUCTION

Why Do I Need This Test?

Electromyography (EMG) tests analyze nerve and muscle electrical activity. Nerve conduction studies are often performed along with an EMG, which is why we discuss them together. Doctors typically order an EMG and nerve conduction tests when people have symptoms of weakness and examination shows impaired muscle strength.

What Will the Results Tell Me?

Muscle tissue is normally electrically quiet at rest. After the needle is inserted, there will be some electrical activity, which will quiet down if the muscle is healthy. At that point the doctor will not see any action potential (part of the process that occurs when neurons fire) on the oscilloscope. When a muscle is contracted voluntarily, action potentials begin to appear.

Abnormal results of an EMG can be caused by disorders and conditions that include but are not limited to herniated disc, amyotrophic lateral sclerosis (ALS), myasthenia gravis, paralysis, spinal stenosis, inflamed muscles, and muscular dystrophy. Abnormal results of a nerve conduction study may indicate carpal tunnel syndrome, Guillain-Barré syndrome, and help find the source of numbness, tingling, and/or pain. Both tests can be used to detect post-polio syndrome.

How Do I Prepare for the Test?
No special preparations are necessary. Do not use any lotions or creams on your skin the day of the test.

What Happens During the Test?
For the EMG, the doctor inserts very thin needles into the muscles being tested. Each needle is attached to a wire that sends signals to a machine. The needles detect electrical patterns inside the muscle and the nerves that are attached to that muscle. Most people say this test is mildly uncomfortable. EMG testing typically takes 20–30 minutes.

For the nerve conduction studies, small pads are taped to the skin on your hands or feet. The pads can deliver mild electric shocks and detect electric signals that come through the skin. You may feel your muscles twitch when an electrical signal is delivered. These studies may take about 30 minutes.

What Happens After the Test?
You can return to your regular activities immediately after the tests. Your muscles may feel sore and/or bruised for a day or two.

What Are the Risks?
There are no risks associated with the EMG or the nerve conduction tests. The EMG needles are tiny and pose no significant risk of infection or bleeding. The electrical shocks are too mild to cause any damage.

EXERCISE STRESS TEST
Why Do I Need This Test?
The exercise stress test, which is also known as the exercise tolerance test or treadmill test, is one of the best tools for diagnosing heart disease. It indicates whether your heart is receiving a sufficient amount of blood and oxygen when it's pumping its hardest. Exercise stress tests are often given to people who have experienced chest pain or other symptoms of coronary artery disease.

Exercise stress tests are also used to evaluate the effectiveness of treatment for heart disease and may be helpful in estimating the risk of disease in people who don't have symptoms but who have risk factors, such as high cholesterol. If you are older than 40 and have risk factors for coronary artery disease, such as high blood pressure or you smoke, ask your doctor whether you need this test.

What Will the Results Tell Me?
The results of an exercise stress test can strongly indicate the presence of coronary artery disease if you experienced symptoms such as chest discomfort, dizziness, or shortness of breath during the test, and these symptoms were accompanied by signs on your EKG that there was inadequate blood flow.

If you experience chest discomfort during the test but your EKG does not show any changes, or vice versa, then the results of the test are inconclusive, although they will still be interpreted as an indication of coronary artery disease. Your doctor may order more tests.

How Do I Prepare for the Test?

You will be most comfortable if you wear loose-fitting clothing and athletic shoes. Make sure you let the doctor who is performing the test know if you have a condition that can affect your ability to take the test, such as arthritis or diabetes (exercise can lower your blood sugar so check your sugar level before the test begins) or if you are taking any medications. Let the testing doctor know if you've experienced any chest pressure or pain on the day of the test. Avoid eating a large meal before the test, as it can make exercising uncomfortable.

What Happens During the Test?

You will undergo an electrocardiogram while lying down and then when standing up, and your blood pressure will be taken. To record your heart's electrical pattern, blood pressure, and heart rate while you exercise on the treadmill, several leads will be taped to your arms and one leg. You will then exercise on the treadmill for about 10 minutes. The person who is monitoring you will change the speed and incline of the treadmill several times while you exercise.

If you experience any chest pain or pressure, shortness of breath, leg pain or weakness, or other symptoms while you are exercise, tell the health-care professionals in the room about them.

A variation of this test is called either a thallium

stress test or MIBI stress test, depending on the radionuclides that are used. The radionuclides allow the clinician to view parts of the heart that are not getting sufficient blood flow.

What Happens After the Test?

You should be able to return to your normal schedule immediately after the test. If your blood pressure rises too high or drops too low during the test, a nurse will check it a few minutes after the test and may continue to monitor your electrocardiogram.

The results usually take several days for your doctor to evaluate.

What Are the Risks?

If you have cardiac disease, you might develop chest pain during the test. If you do, tell the medical staff immediately so they can stop the procedure. An exercise stress test is considered extremely safe if doctors examine their patients before the test to ensure they are healthy enough to take it.

FECAL OCCULT BLOOD TEST
Why Do I Need This Test?

A fecal occult blood test finds blood in stool by placing a small stool sample on a chemically treated card, pad, or cloth wipe. A chemical solution is placed on the sample, and if the card, pad, or cloth turns blue, there is blood in the sample.

Fecal occult blood tests are usually done as part

of a routine examination and as a screening tool for early detection of colorectal cancer. The American Cancer Society and other major health organizations recommend that the test be done yearly starting at age 50 or earlier if ordered by a doctor because of your family history. Your doctor may also order a fecal occult blood test if he or she suspects you have an anemia that might be caused by gastrointestinal bleeding. These tests are often done at home using a home test kit (see "Colorectal Disease Test," in the Home Medical Tests section.).

What Will the Results Tell Me?

A negative test result means no blood was found. A positive test result indicates abnormal bleeding within your gastrointestinal tract. The bleeding may be caused by a variety of problems, including hemorrhoids, anal fissures, colon polyps, peptic ulcers, ulcerative colitis, gastroesophageal reflux disease (GERD), Crohn's disease, or colorectal cancer. It is important to note that although a fecal occult blood test can be used to check for colorectal cancer, it is never used to diagnose it. Other tests for colorectal cancer include a digital rectal examination, flexible sigmoidoscopy, colonoscopy, and CT (computed tomography) scan.

How Do I Prepare For the Test?

See "Colorectal Disease Test" in the Home Medical Tests section.

What Happens During the Test?
See "Colorectal Disease Test" in the Home Medical Tests section.

What Happens After the Test?
See "Colorectal Disease Test" in the Home Medical Tests section.

What are the Risks?
There are no risks associated with the fecal occult blood test.

HIV TEST
Also see "HIV Testing" in the Home Medical Tests section.

Why Do I Need This Test?
The standard HIV test looks for antibodies in your blood. Antibodies are special proteins that the body produces in response to an infection; in this case, the human immunodeficiency virus.

You should have an HIV test if you are sexually active and you have any reason to be unsure about the sexual health of your partner(s). Undergoing HIV testing is the only way to know if you are infected with HIV, as generally there are no symptoms. Getting a negative result will relieve any worry, while a positive result can allow you to take steps to manage the disease and to protect other people. Many people who are HIV-positive stay healthy for many years. If you become ill, there are many drugs (antiretrovirals) that can slow down progression of the virus. Also, knowing your HIV status may have an impact on your future decisions about relationships and having children.

What Will the Results Tell Me?

If you get tested earlier than 3 months after infection, the results may be unclear, as you need to allow up to 90 days for antibodies to HIV to develop. During that time (called the "window period") you may have high levels of HIV in your blood, sexual fluids, or breast milk, and you can transmit the virus to another person even though you do not test positive on an antibody test.

Standard HIV antibody tests are at least 99.5% accurate in detecting HIV antibodies. A negative test result at three months nearly always means you are not infected with HIV. However, depending on whether you have engaged in any risky behavior that could have exposed you to the virus, you may want to do another test in six months.

If you get a positive result, it must be confirmed using a second test. Secondary tests include:

• Western blot assays: the most accurate, but also the most complex to administer

• Indirect immunofluorescence assay: similar to the Western blot, but this one uses a microscope to detect HIV antibodies

- A second standard HIV antibody test: usually used when resources are poor. The second test should be a different commercial brand.

When the results of two tests are combined, the chances of getting an inaccurate result is less than 0.1%.

How Do I Prepare for the Test?
There are no special preparations for the test.

What Happens During the Test?
A health-care professional usually draws the blood from a vein located on the inside of the arm near the elbow. First the skin surface is cleaned with an alcohol pad and an elastic band is placed around the upper arm, which causes the veins to swell with blood. A needle is inserted into a vein and blood is withdrawn by a syringe into a special vacuumed vial. Once the blood has been withdrawn, the elastic band is removed and the collection site is covered with a bandage to stop any bleeding.

Home HIV test kits are also available; see "HIV Testing" in the Home Medical Tests section.

What Happens After the Test?
You should be able to return to your normal routine immediately after the test. However, in some cases individuals feel slightly light-headed for a few minutes after blood is drawn.

What Are the Risks?

An HIV test is considered a very safe procedure. However, there are some problems that may occur when blood is drawn, such as feeling faint or light-headed, development of a hematoma (blood that accumulates under the skin, resulting in a lump or bruise), or pain associated with the health-care professional having to make several attempts at locating a vein.

LIPID PANEL

Why Do I Need This Test?

A lipid panel, also called a lipid profile, is a group of tests that measures the levels of four fats: cholesterol, high-density lipoprotein (HDL), low-density lipoprotein (LDL), and triglycerides. These fats play a significant role in the risk of developing coronary heart disease. A lipid panel can also be used to monitor treatment for high cholesterol and heart disease.

It is recommended that healthy adults who have no risk factors for heart disease undergo a lipid panel every five years. Risk factors include obesity, diabetes, high cholesterol, high triglycerides, high blood pressure, and family history of heart disease, among others. Those who have risk factors should be tested more regularly, as directed by their doctor. Although screening with a lipid profile is not usually ordered for children and adolescents, those who are at an increased risk of developing heart disease as adults should be screened.

What Will the Results Tell Me?

The results of your lipid profile, along with other known risk factors of heart disease, will help you and your doctor determine your risk of developing disease and what treatment, if any, is necessary. Options include lifestyle changes (diet, exercise, stopping smoking, stress management) and medication.

The results of your profile will give you levels in four areas. Here are the goal guidelines that doctors use when determining a patient's risk of heart disease.

- LDL
  - Should be less than 100 mg/dL if you have heart disease or diabetes
  - Less than 130 mg/dL if you have 2 or more risk factors
  - Less than 160 mg/dL if you have 1 or no risk factors

- HDL
  - Less than 40 mg/dL for men and less than 50 mg/dL for women indicates an increased risk of heart disease
  - 40–59 mg/dL for men and 50–59 mg/dL for women is associated with average risk of heart disease

- 60 mg/dL or higher is associated with a less than average risk of heart disease

- Cholesterol
  - Less than 200 mg/dL is optimal. If your LDL, HDL, and triglyceride levels are also at desirable levels and you have no other risk factors for heart disease, you are at relatively low risk of coronary heart disease.
  - 201 to 239 mg/dL is borderline high risk. Your doctor will evaluate your LDL, HDL, and triglyceride levels. It is possible to have borderline high total cholesterol and normal LDL and HDL levels.
  - 240 mg/dL and greater is high cholesterol. Typically people with this high level have twice the risk of coronary heart disease. You and your doctor should establish a prevention and treatment plan.

- Triglycerides
  - Less than 150 mg/dL is normal
  - 150–199 mg/dL is borderline high
  - 200–499 mg/dL is high
  - 500 mg/dL or greater is very high

Some laboratories report a ratio of total cholesterol to HDL cholesterol, which is calculated by dividing the total cholesterol by the HDL cholesterol. This ratio is helpful in determining appropriate treatment. If you have a total cholesterol of 200 mg/dL and an HDL of 50 mg/dL, the ratio would be 4:1. A desirable ratio is lower than 5:1, with an optimal ratio of 3.5:1.

How Do I Prepare for the Test?

Tell your doctor if you are taking any medications on a regular basis, as you may need to stop them for the test. You will be asked to not eat or drink anything except water for 12 hours before the test. Do not take this test if you are ill, as cholesterol is temporarily low during acute illness, immediately following a heart attack, or during stress. If you were recently pregnant, you should wait at least 6 weeks after your baby is born to have your HDL measured.

What Happens During the Test?

A health-care professional usually draws the blood from a vein located on the inside of the arm near the elbow. First the skin surface is cleaned with an alcohol pad and an elastic band is placed around the upper arm, which causes the veins to swell with blood. A needle is inserted into a vein and blood is withdrawn by a syringe into a special vacuumed vial. Once the blood has been withdrawn, the elastic band is removed and the collection site is covered with a bandage to stop any bleeding.

What Happens After the Test?

You should be able to return to your normal routine immediately after the test. However, in some cases

individuals feel slightly light-headed for a few minutes after blood is drawn.

What Are the Risks?
A lipid panel is considered a very safe procedure. However, there are some problems that may occur when
blood is drawn, such as feeling faint or light-headed,
development of a hematoma (blood that accumulates
under the skin, resulting in a lump or bruise), or pain
associated with the health-care professional having to
make several attempts at locating a vein.

LIVER PANEL
Why Do I Need This Test?
A liver panel, which is also known as liver (hepatic)
function tests, is used to detect, evaluate, and monitor
problems with the liver. A doctor usually orders a liver
panel when he or she suspects a liver condition because
of certain symptoms, such as jaundice, dark urine, or
light-colored bowel movements; nausea, vomiting,
and/or diarrhea; loss of appetite; vomiting of blood;
black or bloody stool; unusual weight changes; fatigue
or loss of stamina; or swelling or pain in the belly.

A liver panel usually consists of seven tests that
are done at the same time on a single blood sample.
Each of the tests and what they can tell you is ex-
plained under "What Will the Results Tell Me?"

Liver disease is frequently first detected through
routine blood testing that is done as part of a physical. This testing, called the Comprehensive Meta-

bolic Panel, includes most of the liver panel tests except the direct bilirubin. When liver disease is discovered with a CMP blood test, it may be monitored with follow-up liver panels.

What Will the Results Tell Me?

Each of the seven tests that make up the liver panel can reveal important information for your doctor. Please note that normal ranges can vary from laboratory to laboratory, so the ranges given here may not be those used by your laboratory. The seven tests include:

- Alanine aminotransferase (ALT): enzyme found mainly in the liver. The best test for detecting hepatitis. Normal adult range: 5–60 IU/L (international units/liter)

- Alkaline phosphatase (ALP): Enzyme related to the bile ducts. Levels are often elevated when they are blocked. Normal adult range: 44–147 IU/L

- Aspartate aminotransferase (AST): Enzyme found in the liver, heart, and other muscles in the body. Normal adult range: 10–34 IU/L

- Bilirubin: Two different tests of bilirubin are usually done together, especially if a person has jaundice. Total bilirubin measures all the bilirubin in the blood, while direct bilirubin determines the level that is combined with another compound in the liver. Normal adult range, total bilirubin: 0–1.3 mg/dL

- Albumin: Measures the level of the main protein manufactured by the liver and reveals whether production is adequate. Normal adult range: 3.9–5.0 g/dL (grams/deciliter)

- Total protein: Measures albumin plus all other proteins in the blood, including antibodies, which fight infection. Normal adult range: 6.5–8.2 g/dL

Abnormal results of your liver function tests may indicate a range of problems, depending on which test results are abnormal. Some of the conditions indicated by abnormal liver panel results include cirrhosis, liver cancer, blockage in the liver or gallbladder, hepatitis, fatty liver (steatosis), gallstones, and alcoholic liver disease.

Although these tests are usually done to look for liver problems, the enzymes are produced in other parts of the body as well. That means elevated levels may be caused by diseases or conditions beyond the liver. Therefore your doctor may order more blood tests to find the source of any extra enzyme. Results that are lower than normal are usually not a concern.

How Do I Prepare for the Test?
Because tests that measure protein levels in the blood are not as accurate if you have eaten, you

should not eat or drink anything for at least 8 hours before your test. If you regularly take medications, talk to your doctor to see if you need to stop any of them before the test.

What Happens During the Test?

A health-care professional will collect a small amount of blood from a vein on the inside of your arm. Usually an elastic band is placed around the top of the arm, which makes the veins prominent. An alcohol pad will be used to wipe the needle insertion area and a needle will be placed into a vein. A syringe will withdraw the blood into a vial, the needle and elastic band will be removed, and a bandage will be placed over the insertion site to stop any bleeding.

What Happens After the Test?

You should be able to return to your regular activities immediately after the test. Occasionally a blood draw causes individuals to feel slightly light-headed for a few minutes after the test is over.

What Are the Risks?

Drawing blood for a liver panel is considered a very safe procedure. However, there are some problems that may occur when blood is drawn, such as feeling faint or light-headed, development of a hematoma (blood that accumulates under the skin, resulting in a lump or bruise), or pain associated with the health-care professional having to make several attempts at locating a vein.

MAMMOGRAM

Why Do I Need This Test?

A mammogram is an X-ray of the breast. Two types of mammograms are done. A screening mammogram is performed to detect breast changes in women who have no signs or symptoms of breast cancer. Typically two X-rays of each breast are taken. A diagnostic mammogram is done to check for breast cancer after a lump or other signs or symptoms (e.g., change in breast size or shape, nipple discharge, skin thickening, pain) of breast cancer have been detected. A diagnostic mammogram involves taking more X-rays to get views of the breasts from several angles.

A diagnostic mammogram is sometimes used to evaluate changes found during a screening mammogram or to see breast tissue that can be difficult to view because of breast implants.

The National Cancer Institute recommends that women age 40 and older have a screening mammogram every 1–2 years. Women who are at high risk of breast cancer are usually encouraged to have a mammogram at an earlier age and should talk to their health-care professional about how often a mammogram should be scheduled.

What Will the Results Tell Me?

Mammograms make it possible to detect breast cancer, benign tumors, and cysts that cannot be felt during a physical examination of the breasts. They can also find tiny calcium deposits (microcalcifications), which sometimes indicate breast cancer. Generally, a regular, well-outlined spot on your X-rays is more likely to be a noncancerous lesion such as a cyst, while a poorly outlined, cloudy area suggests breast cancer. Doctors may perform a biopsy if the mammogram looks suspicious to determine if the abnormality is cancerous or noncancerous.

The recent introduction of digital mammography promises better breast images because they can be enhanced by computer technology. This is especially helpful for women who have dense breast tissue.

How Do I Prepare for the Test?

Before the mammogram, tell your doctor if you are pregnant or suspect you may be pregnant, if you are breastfeeding, or if you have breast implants. You may be asked to sign a consent form before having the test. Do not apply any deodorant, powder, ointments, or perfumes in the underarm and breast area on the day of the test, as they can interfere with the results.

What Happens During the Test?

You will be asked to remove clothing from your waist up and be given a gown to wear. You must also remove any jewelry or other objects that might interfere with the test. You will stand in front of a mammography machine and one breast will be placed on the X-ray plate. The technologist may place an adhesive marker if you have any moles or other spots that might interfere with the image.

A second flat plate will be lowered over your

breast and compress it against the X-ray plate. You may feel some temporary discomfort while your breast is being pressed. The technologist will ask you to hold your breath while the images are taken. After both breasts have been X-rayed, the technologist will ask you to wait while a radiologist examines the films to make sure they are clear. If any of the images are of questionable quality, you may be asked to have another image or two taken.

What Happens After the Test?
You may return to your regular activities right after the mammogram is done.

What Are the Risks?
Mammography involves a very low dose of radiation. Scientific research shows that doses 100–1,000 times greater than those used during mammography are necessary to show any statistical increase in breast cancer frequency.

PAPANICOLAOU TEST
Why Do I Need This Test?
The Papanicolaou test, or Pap smear, is an evaluation of a sample of cells from the cervix. This test is primarily used to check for cervical cancer, but it can also test for human papillomavirus, or HPV. Although cervical cancer is caused by infection with HPV, only a fraction of women who have HPV get

cervical cancer. Early detection of cervical cancer gives you a greater chance at a cure. A Pap smear can also identify changes in cervical cells that suggest cancer may develop in the future.

A Pap smear is usually done along with a pelvic examination, during which the doctor examines a woman's external genitals, vagina, uterus, ovaries, and rectum. Although a pelvic examination can screen for problems with the reproductive organs, only a Pap smear can detect early cervical cancer or precancers.

All women who are 21 or older, and younger women who are sexually active, should have a Pap smear every 1–3 years. It should be done more often if any of the smears have detected abnormalities or if you have certain risk factors. Therefore, regardless of age a woman should have a Pap smear every year if she has:

- Ever had precancerous cells or a diagnosis of cervical cancer

- Been exposed to diethylstilbestrol before birth

- HIV infection

- A weakened immune system because of chemotherapy, an organ transplant, or corticosteroid use

What Will the Results Tell Me?

It can take 1–2 weeks to get your test results. If the cervical cells are normal, the result is said to be negative. If the test shows abnormal or unusual cells, the result is positive. A positive result means abnormal cells were found, but it does not necessarily mean you have cancer. Here are some of the things your doctor may find:

- Atypical squamous cells of undetermined significance: Squamous cells are flat, thin cells that grow on the surface of a healthy cervix. If abnormal cells are found, your doctor can reanalyze the sample to look for viruses that are known to promote the development of cancer. If no high-risk viruses are found, the abnormal cells seen in your original test are likely not of concern.

- Squamous intraepithelial lesion: These cells may be precancerous. If the cell changes (in size, shape, and other characteristics) are low-grade, and if a precancerous lesion is present, the development of cancer is likely years away. If the changes are high-grade, there is a greater chance that the lesion may turn into cancer sooner. Your doctor will probably order more tests.

- Atypical glandular cells: These cells may appears to be abnormal, but further testing will be needed to determine their source and if they are significant.

- Squamous cancer or adenocarcinoma cells: These cells appear to be so abnormal that the presence of cancer is almost certain. Squamous refers to cancers that develop in the flat surface cells of the cervix or vagina, while adenocarcinoma refers to cancers that occur in glandular cells. Your doctor will recommend an immediate evaluation.

Any abnormal finding on a Pap smear may prompt your doctor to perform a procedure called colposcopy, which uses a special magnifying device (colposcope) to examine the tissues of the cervix, vagina, and vulva. A colposcopy may include a biopsy taken from any areas that have abnormal cells.

How Do I Prepare for the Test?
A Pap smear should be done when you are not experiencing menstrual bleeding. You should not douche, use a tampon, or have intercourse for 24 hours before the test. Do not use any vaginal creams on the day of your test.

What Happens During the Test?
Your doctor may ask you to undress completely or simply from the waist down and to put on a gown. You will lie on your back on an exam table with your knees bent and with your heels resting in supports

called stirrups. The doctor will use an instrument called a speculum to hold the walls of your vagina apart so he or she can insert a cotton swab or spatula to collect cell samples from the cervix. The speculum may feel cold and cause a feeling of pressure in your pelvic area. You may feel some slight cramping when the doctor collects the cells, but otherwise the procedure is painless. The doctor will then transfer the cell sample to a slide for examination under a microscope.

What Happens After the Test?
You can return to your regular activities immediately after the test. Some women experience a small amount of spotting after the test.

What are the Risks?
There are no risks associated with this test.

PROSTATE-SPECIFIC ANTIGEN TEST
Why Do I Need This Test?
The prostate-specific antigen (PSA) test measures the amount of this antigen in the blood. Prostate-specific antigen is made by the prostate by both normal and cancer cells. The PSA test is used mainly to screen for prostate cancer, but it also can be used to identify benign prostatic hyperplasia (BPH), a noncancerous enlargement of the prostate gland; and prostatitis, an infection or inflammation of the prostate gland.

Currently, Medicare provides coverage for an annual PSA test for all men age 50 and older. Many doctors recommend that men who are at a higher risk for prostate cancer begin screening at age 40 or 45. Although nearly 65 percent of prostate cancer cases occur in men who are age 65 or older, other risk factors include a family history of the disease, race (African American men have the highest rate; Asian and Native American men have the lowest), and possibly a high-fat diet. Early detection of prostate cancer allows you and your doctor time to establish a treatment strategy.

What Can the Results Tell Me?

The results report the level of PSA detected in the blood as nanograms of PSA per milliliter (ng/mL) of blood. At one time most doctors considered PSA values less than 4.0 ng/mL to be normal. However, recent research has found prostate cancer in men with PSA levels below 4.0 ng/mL. The following ranges are now used as a guideline, with individual variation:

- 0 to 2.5 ng/mL is low

- 2.6 to 10 ng/mL is slightly to moderately elevated

- 10 to 19.9 ng/mL is moderately elevated

- 20 ng/mL or higher is significantly elevated

The higher the PSA level, the more likely it is that cancer is present. However, one abnormal PSA test result does not necessarily mean a man has cancer nor that more diagnostic tests are required. Elevated PSA test results can also indicate benign prostate enlargement, inflammation, and infection. Age affects PSA levels, and ranges vary somewhat from laboratory to laboratory. When having repeat PSA tests done, the same laboratory should be used so a reliable comparison of the results can be made.

If PSA test results increase over several testing times or if a lump is detected during a physical examination, the doctor may order other tests to determine if cancer or another problem is the cause. A urinalysis can detect a urinary tract infection, while imaging tests (e.g., ultrasound, X-rays, cystoscopy) can detect stones or other abnormalities. If cancer is suspected, a biopsy is necessary to identify whether the cancer has affected the prostate.

How Do I Prepare for the Test?

Because ejaculation can cause PSA levels to rise for a short time before they go down again, doctors typically recommend that men refrain from ejaculation for two days before the test. Also, tell your doctor about any medications you are taking, as some can lower PSA levels. Some herbal remedies can also impact PSA and mask high levels.

What Happens During the Test?

A health-care professional usually draws the blood from a vein located on the inside of the arm near the elbow. First the skin surface is cleaned with an alcohol pad and an elastic band is placed around the upper arm, which causes the veins to swell with blood. A needle is inserted into a vein and blood is withdrawn by a syringe or a connection into a special vacuumed vial. Once the blood has been withdrawn, the elastic band is removed and the collection site is covered with a bandage to stop any bleeding. The sample is then analyzed in a laboratory.

What Happens After the Test?

You should be able to return to your regular activities immediately after the test. However, some individuals experience mild light-headedness after a blood draw.

What Are the Risks?

Having blood drawn for a PSA test is considered a very safe procedure. However, there are some problems that may occur when blood is drawn, such as feeling faint or light-headed, development of a hematoma (blood that accumulates under the skin, resulting in a lump or bruise), or pain associated with the health-care professional having to make several attempts at locating a vein.

PULMONARY FUNCTION TEST
Why Do I Need This Test?

Pulmonary function testing can reveal a great deal of information about your lungs and lung function. Your doctor may order the testing if you smoke, if you are experiencing shortness of breath or other breathing difficulties, or if there is suspicion of a pulmonary condition such as asthma, emphysema, or chronic obstructive pulmonary disease. The tests can tell your doctor the quantity of air you breathe, how well your lungs deliver oxygen to your blood, and how efficiently you move air in and out of your lungs. Pulmonary function testing can also help your doctor monitor your lung function if you are regularly exposed to substances that can damage your lungs.

What Will the Results Tell Me?

The normal value ranges for pulmonary function tests will be adjusted for your age, sex, and height, and sometimes for weight and race. Results are given as a percentage of the expected value, and they are usually available right after the tests are completed.

Normal test results are those that are within the range for people with healthy lungs. Abnormal results may indicate either obstructive or restrictive lung disease. Obstructive lung disease is any condition in which the airways are narrowed. This can be caused by conditions such as asthma, infection (which involves inflammation), bronchitis, or emphysema.

Restrictive lung disease involves a loss of lung

tissue, a reduction in the ability of the lungs to expand, or a decrease in the ability of the lungs to transfer oxygen to the blood. Restrictive lung disease can be caused by various conditions, such as pneumonia, sarcoidosis, scleroderma, pulmonary fibrosis, obesity, or chest injury.

How Do I Prepare for the Test?

Tell your doctor if you are taking any medications, especially for lung problems such as asthma. You may need to stop taking some medications before the test. Also let your doctor know if you have had a recent heart attack or chest pains.

Do not eat a heavy meal right before the test because a full stomach makes it difficult to fully expand your lungs. Avoid drinks and food that contain caffeine for 24 hours before the test. Do not smoke or exercise strenuously for 6 hours before the test.

What Happens During the Test?

This testing is usually done in a special laboratory by a respiratory therapist. During the tests, you will breathe in and out through a tube that is connected to various devices. One test is spirometry, which measures how forcefully you can inhale and exhale. Another measures lung volume in one of two ways. You may be asked to inhale a small amount of a specific gas (e.g., helium), which mixes with the air in your lungs before you are asked to exhale. When you exhale, the air and helium will be calculated to see how much air your lungs were holding. The other way to measure lung volume is called plethysmography. In this test, you sit inside an airtight room and breathe in and out through a tube in the wall. This test measures pressure change and is used to calculate the amount of air you breathe.

Another test measures diffusion capacity, which is the ability to absorb gases, including oxygen. To measure this, you inhale a small amount of carbon monoxide and the amount you exhale is measured.

If you have indications of asthma, your doctor may also include the inhalation challenge test, which measures the response of your airways to substances (allergens) that may be causing your symptoms. During this test, increasing amounts of an allergen are inhaled through a nebulizer. Before and after you inhale the substances, spirometry readings are taken to evaluate your lung function.

You may undergo variations of any of these tests, depending on what your doctor orders. If you feel pain or discomfort at any time during the tests, tell the technician immediately.

What Happens After the Test?

You can return to your regular activities immediately after the test is done. Some people feel tired after the tests, especially if they have lung disease.

What Are the Risks?

There are no risks associated with the test.

SKIN BIOPSY

Why Do I Need This Test?

Skin biopsies are taken to diagnose growths such as skin cancers (skin cancer is the most common cancer in the United States), precancerous cells, keratoses, or inflammatory skin disorders such as psoriasis and contact dermatitis. The most widely used technique for skin biopsy is the punch biopsy, and it can be performed for both diagnostic and therapeutic purposes, as when it is used to remove warts, skin cancers, moles, or other growths. Recently it has been used to help predict or diagnose diabetic neuropathy in high-risk patients.

Early diagnosis of abnormal skin lesions and biopsy can help identify skin cancers and lead to early treatment.

What Will the Results Tell Me?

If the tissue sample is benign, no further action may be necessary. Noncancerous skin changes can include skin tags, warts, seborrheic keratoses, keloids, and benign tumors such as neurofibromas or dermatofibromas.

If the biopsy reveals cancer, the microscopic examination can identify the type of malignant cells and your physician can make plans to completely remove the cells. The presence of cells that are involved in inflammation can help your doctor diagnose the disease, which may include lupus, psoriasis, or vasculitis, among others. When trying to diagnose inflammation, your doctor may need to take another skin sample when the condition reaches another stage of development because inflammatory diseases can appear in various ways. If the results of a biopsy are inconclusive, your doctor may order another biopsy.

How Do I Prepare for the Test?
There is no special preparation for a skin biopsy. However, do tell your doctor if you have a known allergy to lidocaine or any related local anesthesia, if you are taking any medications (especially anti-inflammatory or blood-thinning drugs), or if you have bleeding problems.

What Happens During the Test?
A skin biopsy is done in a doctor's office, usually by a dermatologist. The health-care provider begins by injecting a local anesthetic (usually with lidocaine) near the sample site. After the initial sting from the injection, the rest of the procedure is painless. The doctor then uses a disposable or sterilized punch to biopsy the lesion or area of skin in question. For non-facial lesions, a 4-mm punch is usually chosen. For conditions that have atypical features or that are granulomatous, a 5-mm punch is commonly used.

The doctor stretches the skin taut and pushes the punch into the skin using a rotating movement. The wound that remains once the biopsy sample is taken can be sutured with one or two stitches, although suturing is optional.

What Happens After the Test?

A dressing and often an antibiotic ointment will be placed on the biopsy site. You may be instructed to clean the site, reapply ointment, and change the dressing once or several times a day until the site heals. This may take up to 28 days, depending on the size and location of the biopsy. It is best not to let the wound dry out, because a scab will delay healing. The site may be sore or bleed slightly for several days.

You can return to your normal schedule immediately after the test. A pathologist will examine the sample under a high-powered microscope and your doctor will report the results to you. Results are usually ready within seven days.

What Are the Risks?

There is a very slight risk of infection and/or of persistent bleeding after a skin biopsy. If you care for the biopsy site as recommended by your doctor, you should experience no problems. If you have excessive bleeding or drainage through the bandage, apply pressure to the site and contact your doctor. Also contact your doctor if you experience increased tenderness, pain, or swelling at the biopsy site, or if you develop a fever.

THYROID NUCLEAR MEDICINE TEST
Why Do I Need This Test?

There are two types of thyroid nuclear medicine tests—a thyroid scan and a radioactive iodine uptake test. Both evaluate the health of the thyroid, and both involve receiving a small amount of a weak radioactive substance called radionuclide.

A thyroid scan can help evaluate inflammation or growths, or investigate the cause of an overactive thyroid. It is typically ordered when a physical examination or laboratory finding indicates that the thyroid is enlarged. A radioactive iodine uptake test measures the amount of radioactivity in your thyroid after you've taken a radioactive iodine pill. The amount of radioactive iodine detected by the test corresponds with the amount of hormone your thyroid is producing.

What Will the Results Tell Me?

A thyroid scan shows the shape, outline, and position of your thyroid so your doctor can determine whether it is enlarged or there are any abnormal growths. It can also provide an estimate of your thyroid activity, although this should be confirmed with a radioactive iodine uptake test. Your doctor should receive a report within a day or two of your test.

Uptake test results are available at the time of the testing, but because follow-up readings need to be compared, your doctor may take several days to report to you. Your doctor is looking for an uptake value, which is the net result of how much iodine your thyroid picked up, how much converted to hormone, and how much either leaked or was secreted into the bloodstream. A low radioactivity reading indicates that your thyroid retained only a small amount of iodine, which suggests the gland is not producing excess hormone but is inflamed and unable to store it. A high reading suggests that your thyroid is overactive, or producing excessive amounts of thyroid hormone.

How Do I Prepare for the Test?

If you may be pregnant, know you are pregnant, or are breast-feeding, tell your doctor before the test. The radionuclides can harm your fetus or nursing infant, so your doctor will need to use an alternative method to diagnose the problem. For about seven days before a thyroid scan, your doctor may ask you to avoid certain foods and medications that can interfere with the test, including shellfish and thyroid hormones. If you will be taking a radioactive iodine uptake test, you also may be asked to fast for several hours before the test so you can take the radioactive iodine pill.

What Happens During the Test?

You may have either one or both thyroid tests at the same time. For a thyroid scan, you will likely recline on a comfortable table with the area around your neck and upper chest clear so the images can be taken. A technician will place a radioactivity detector (a specially designed camera) against your neck and take several images. The camera does not emit any radiation. A thyroid scan takes about 30 minutes.

If you undergo the iodine reuptake test, it can be done while you sit. A technician will place a probe several inches in front of your neck and measure the percentage of radioactivity that is being retained by your thyroid. You will need to return within approximately 24 hours for follow-up testing to get a second set of readings. These will be compared with the first set to identify how much hormone has been formed and secreted.

What Happens After the Test?

You can return to your regular activities immediately after the test. Nearly all of the weakly radioactive substances taken during these tests are eliminated from the body within a day or two. Even during that time, however, they pose no danger to you or anyone else.

What Are the Risks?

The amount of radiation involved with these tests is comparable to that from a routine X-ray, and the amount of radionuclide administered is minuscule and unlikely to cause allergic reactions or side effects.

THYROID PANEL
Why Do I Need This Test?

The thyroid panel, also known as thyroid hormone testing, is a group of tests used to evaluate thyroid function and to help diagnose thyroid disorders. The tests measure the amount of thyroid hormones in your blood. The panel usually includes:

- TSH (thyroid-stimulating hormone, or thyrotropin): Measured to test for hypothyroidism, hyperthyroidism and to monitor thyroid replacement therapy. TSH screening is performed routinely on newborns as part of each state's newborn screening program. It can also be used to diagnose and monitor female infertility problems

- T4 or free T4 (thyroxine): Test for hypothyroidism and hyperthyroidism

- T3 or free T3 (triiodothyronine): Test for hyperthyroidism

Your doctor may order a thyroid panel if you have signs and symptoms of hyperthyroidism or hypothyroidism, or if your thyroid gland is enlarged. The American Thyroid Association recommends that adults older than age 35 undergo thyroid screening every 5 years, although not all experts agree with this recommendation. Some organizations do recommend that women older than 50 or who are at high risk for thyroid disorders get screened every few years.

What Will the Results Tell Me?

A low TSH can indicate hyperthyroidism or excessive amounts of thyroid hormone medication if you are being treated for hypothyroidism. A high TSH and normal T4 and T3 indicate mild hypothyroidism, while high TSH, low T4, and low or normal T3 is stronger for hypothyroidism. Low TSH along with high or normal T4 and high or normal T3 is an indication of hyperthyroidism. Rarely, a high TSH value indicates that the pituitary gland is malfunctioning, perhaps producing unregulated levels of the hormone due to a tumor.

How Do I Prepare for the Test?

Medications such as aspirin and thyroid-hormone replacement therapy may affect the results of a thyroid panel, so tell your doctor about any drugs you are taking before you take the test. Other factors that can affect test results include extreme stress, acute illness, and pregnancy.

What Happens During the Test?

A health-care professional usually draws the blood from a vein located on the inside of the arm near the elbow. First the skin surface is cleaned with an alcohol pad and an elastic band is placed around the upper arm, which causes the veins to swell with blood. A needle is inserted into a vein and blood is withdrawn by a syringe into a special vacuumed vial. Once the blood has been withdrawn, the elastic band is removed and the collection site is covered with a bandage to stop any bleeding.

What Happens After the Test?

You should be able to return to your normal routine immediately after the test. However, in some cases individuals feel slightly light-headed for a few minutes after blood is drawn.

What Are the Risks?

A thyroid panel is considered a very safe procedure. However, there are some problems that may occur when blood is drawn, such as feeling faint or light-headed, development of a hematoma (blood that accumulates under the skin, resulting in a lump or bruise), or pain associated with the health-care professional having to make several attempts at locating a vein.

TONOMETRY

Why Do I Need This Test?

Tonometry is a test that measures the amount of pressure in your eyeballs, which is called intraocular pressure (IOP). High pressure inside the eye is caused by glaucoma, a disease that can damage your optic nerve and cause blindness if it is not treated. Damage to the optic nerve can result when an accumulation of fluid in the eye does not drain properly.

Since glaucoma is a very common vision problem, it is recommended that all adults older than age 40 have tonometry every 3–5 years to check for the disease. Tonometry is also helpful for monitoring the effectiveness of any medications you are taking for glaucoma.

What Will The Results Tell Me?

Results of the test will tell you if you have excessive IOP levels and if you are developing glaucoma. Tonometry tests may be done over months or years to check for glaucoma, as the buildup of pressure can occur very gradually. If your IOP is high, your doctor will likely order more tests, such as ophthalmoscopy (allows the doctor to see the back of the eye), gonioscopy (allows the doctor to see the front part of the eye between the cornea and the iris), and visual field testing (various factors are checked, including near and far distances, gaps in vision, and colors).

How Do I Prepare for the Test?

You will need to remove contact lenses if you wear them. Also tell your doctor if you have any type of eye infection or eye problem. Results from tonometry will be most accurate if you do not drink more than 16 ounces of fluid 4 hours before the test, do not drink alcohol for 12 hours before the test, and do not smoke marijuana for 24 hours before the test.

What Happens During the Test?

There are several tonometry methods your doctor may use. Regardless of the method used, your chin will sit in a padded support while you stare straight ahead so the doctor can do the test.

- Air-puff tonometry (pneumotonometry). This is a noncontact form of tonometry that uses a puff of air to flatten the cornea. It is not the most accurate way to measure IOP, but it often used because it is simple and is the easiest way to test children. It is also used for people who have had laser-assisted in-situ keratomileusis (LASIK) surgery. No numbing eyedrops are needed. The doctor shines a bright light into your eyes and a brief puff of air is blown at your eye. You will feel mild pressure or coolness on your eye. The test can be repeated several times for each eye.

- Applanation tonometry: In this method, the doctor first puts eye-numbing eyedrops into your eyes and a dye (fluorescein) applied either by touching a strip of treated paper to your eye, or the dye will be in the eyedrops. The dye makes it easier for the doctor to see your cornea. Then he or she gently flattens the cornea with a small probe to measure IOP and uses a microscope to examine your eyes. This approach is very accurate and is

usually used to measure IOP after a screening test (e.g., air-puff tonometry) has found
increased IOP.

• Electronic indentation tonometry: This approach is being used more often to identify
increased IOP because it is very accurate.
After applying eye-numbing eyedrops, the
doctor gently places the rounded tip of a
penlike instrument on your cornea. Four
readings are taken on each eye. Each time
an accurate reading occurs, you will hear a
beeping sound. The IOP results show on a
computer panel.

You may feel like blinking during the test, but the
test is painless.

What Happens After the Test?
If you wear contact lenses, do not put them back in
until 2 hours after the test. Until that time you can
wear eyeglasses if you have them. If you received
eye-numbing eyedrops, do not rub your eyes for at
least 30 minutes after the test.

What Are the Risks?
There is a very slight risk that the doctor may scratch
your cornea if contact tonometry is done. Also, if you
rub your eyes before the anesthesia wear off, you increase the risk of scratching the cornea. A scratched

cornea is uncomfortable but it normally heals in about 24 hours.

Rarely, people have an allergic reaction to the eyedrops used to numb the eyes.

URINALYSIS
Why Do I Need This Test?
Doctors usually order a urinalysis when there is a suspicion of a urinary tract infection or other health problem that can cause abnormalities in the urine, such as cloudiness, brown color, and presence of blood. A urinalysis can measure the number and variety of red and white blood cells, the presence of bacteria and other substances foreign to the urine (e.g., glucose, proteins), the pH of the urine, and the concentration of the urine.

What Will the Results Tell Me?
If a urinalysis shows white blood cells and bacteria, this indicates an infection of the kidneys or bladder. Your doctor may send the sample to a lab for a culture to identify the bacteria that are causing the infection, or simply prescribe an antibiotic to treat the infection. Determination of urinary pH is helpful in the diagnosis and treatment of urinary tract infections and calculi (hard lumps composed of concentrated mineral salts). The presence of red blood cells in urine (hematuria) can indicate dozens of conditions, including glomerulonephritis,

polycystic kidney disease, prostatitis, and tuberculosis.

If the results show excess protein in the urine (proteinuria), it may indicate renal disease or any one of several dozen other conditions, including the use of nonsteroidal anti-inflammatory drugs. Excess glucose in the urine (glycosuria) is an indication of diabetes, liver disease, pancreatic disease, and Cushing's syndrome.

How Do I Prepare for the Test?
There is no special preparation required. Tell your doctor about any medications or supplements you are taking, as some can affect the appearance of urine. A day or two before the test, refrain from eating carrots, beets, blackberries, and rhubarb, as these foods can color the urine.

What Happens During the Test?
In most cases, urine is collected in a clean container, such as a plastic cup, which a nurse or other healthcare professional may give to you. The goal is to get a clean-catch midstream sample. This means you should clean the genital area, urinate a small amount into the toilet, stop, and then urinate again into the collection container.

What Happens After the Test?
You can return to your regular activities. If you have been asked to take a urine sample at home and bring

it to a lab or doctor's office, you should refrigerate the sample after collection.

What Are the Risks?
There are no risks associated with urinalysis.

CHAPTER 3

HOME MEDICAL TESTS

Are you worried about high cholesterol? Do you think you might be pregnant? Do you suspect you are allergic to mold or dust mites but don't want to go to a doctor for the test? Do you want to keep tabs on your blood sugar levels at home?

Then you may want to try a home medical test kit. Home medical kits have been on the market for more than 30 years, when home pregnancy test kits and blood-sugar tests for diabetes were introduced. Today there are several dozen test kits and/or home test devices available over the counter.

Home medical test kits and devices allow you to gather some basic health information at home. In most cases you have results within minutes, although some tests require you to send a sample to a laboratory and you must wait for results. Generally, using home tests sure beats making an appointment with a doctor or clinic and then waiting a week or more for the visit, then waiting longer for the test and finally the results.

Home medical tests can't screen for or diagnose all health problems, but you may be surprised at the number of tests that are now available at your local pharmacy, health-food store, big-box stores, and on-line. Just because they are available, however, does not mean that they are all accurate or safe. Here are some guidelines you should follow when considering use of a home medical test kit.

- Do not use a home test kit to diagnose a medical condition. For example, you should not use a home glucose monitor to diagnose yourself with diabetes: you should see your doctor about getting a fasting blood sugar test and perhaps other blood work to make that determination. If you take a home pregnancy test and it comes out positive, you should see your doctor for an examination and confirmation of your pregnancy.

- Read the instructions. This is probably the number one mistake people make, and the one that can lead to inaccurate results. Do not assume you know how to conduct any home test; always read the instructions.

- Only purchase test kits that have been approved by the Food and Drug Administration (FDA).

- Talk to your physician about your test results. Although a test may have FDA approval, false negatives and false positives can still occur.

- Always check the expiration date. If it has passed, don't buy or use the test.

- Do not change your current medication schedule based on the results of a home test. Talk to your doctor first.

- Look for any warnings or precautions listed on the test kit label. The instructions may ask you to avoid certain foods, medications, alcohol, or physical activity before using the test. If you have any questions, call your doctor or the test manufacturer.

ALLERGY TEST
Why Do I Need This Test?
This test can be convenient for anyone who is experiencing symptoms such as sneezing, runny nose, watery eyes, and headaches and wants to know whether they are caused by an allergy. Knowing what to treat is your first step to feeling better. Once you identify your allergen(s), you can take the proper steps to reduce or eliminate your symptoms.

How Do I Use This Test?

The home allergy test contains finger stick lancets, a blood collection tube, alcohol pad, adhesive bandage, personal information and registration cards, and mailing supplies.

You should use the alcohol pad to wipe the finger you will stick with the lancet. Place four to five drops of blood into the collection tube and seal it. Use the adhesive bandage to cover the stick site. Then place your blood sample into the self-addressed mailer. Once the lab receives your test, you will receive an e-mail directing you to the company's Web site so you can view, download, and print your test results. Your information is secure because you will have a unique patient identification number included in your test kit. You can also get your results by U.S. mail.

What Will the Results Tell Me?

The home allergy test kit can identify ten of the most common allergens, including cat, dust mites, mold, eggs, wheat, milk, and four common airborne allergens—Bermuda grass, mountain cedar (juniper), short ragweed, and timothy grass. It is also possible that you are allergic to other substances not included in this study. For those you will need to see your doctor.

BLOOD PRESSURE TEST
Why Do I Need This Test?

A home blood pressure test allows you to monitor your pressure easily at home, either daily or at whatever interval you and your doctor decide upon. According to the American Heart Association, more than 73 million adults in the United States have high blood pressure (hypertension), and about one quarter of them don't even know it. Even among those who know they have hypertension, about 69 percent are under treatment and 54 percent do not have their pressure under control.

High blood pressure usually has no symptoms, and because it can place you at risk for so many serious problems, it is important for you to know what your pressure is. Some of those problems include atherosclerosis, stroke, heart disease, kidney disease, eye disease (hypertensive retinopathy), diabetes, erectile dysfunction, and preeclampsia. When high blood pressure does have symptoms, they may include nausea, headache, dizziness, and blurred vision, which are common complaints and so can easily be overlooked.

The American Heart Association recommends that people with hypertension or suspected high blood pressure should routinely self-monitor. Included in this recommendation are older people and those who experience "white-coat hypertension," a spike in blood pressure when they are tested by a doctor or other medical professional. By taking an active role in monitoring your blood pressure, you can take more control of your health.

How Do I Use This Test?

It is recommended that you not eat, use tobacco products, exercise, or take medications known to raise blood pressure for at least 30 minutes before you take your blood pressure. You should also avoid taking your pressure if you are upset or nervous: rest for about 15 minutes before attempting the test.

You should take your blood pressure while you are seated in a comfortable position. Your arm should be slightly bent and resting on a table so that your upper arm is on the same level as your heart. Expose your upper arm by rolling up your sleeve, removing your shirt, or slipping your arm out of the sleeve.

Do not move or talk while you are taking your blood pressure. Blood pressure readings can vary 10 to 20 mmHg (millimeters of mercury) between your right and left arms, so it is best to always use the same arm for readings. Blood pressure also varies throughout the day: readings are typically highest in the morning after you get up, decline during the day, and are lowest in the evening.

The instructions for using a blood pressure monitor vary depending on the type of device. Here are some general guidelines. Please carefully read the instructions that come with your monitor and ask your doctor or other health-care professional to help you if you have any questions. It is a good idea to have a professional watch you use your monitor at first so you can be sure you are using it properly.

There are two main types of blood pressure monitors you can use at home. One is a **manual model**, which includes an arm cuff that is connected to a gauge, a squeeze bulb that inflates the cuff, a stethoscope, and a gauge that indicates the blood pressure. To use a manual model, place the cuff around your upper arm so that the lower edge of the cuff is about 1 inch above the bend of your elbow.

Locate the artery on the inside of your elbow by feeling for a pulse with your fingers. Place the earpieces of the stethoscope in your ears and the bell of the stethoscope over the pulse, just below the cuff. It is important to correctly position the stethoscope because the accuracy of your blood pressure reading depends on it.

Close the valve on the inflating bulb, then squeeze the bulb rapidly with your opposite hand to inflate the cuff. Keep squeezing the bulb until the dial reads about 30 mmHg higher than your usual systolic (upper number) pressure. If you do not know your usual pressure, inflate the cuff to 210 mmHg.

Open the pressure valve just enough to allow the pressure to decline gradually, about 2–3 mmHg per second. As the pressure falls, note the number at which you first hear a tapping or pulsing sound through the stethoscope. This number is your systolic blood pressure.

Continue to let the air out. When the sounds finally disappear, note the number on the gauge. This is your diastolic blood pressure. Now you can release all the remaining air in the cuff.

Automatic (or electronic) blood pressure monitors are easier to use and becoming very common and inexpensive. They are battery operated and consist of a cuff that is connected to an electronic monitor that automatically inflates and deflates the cuff. To begin, press the on/off button on the monitor and wait for the heart symbol to appear on the display screen. Then press Start. The cuff will inflate automatically to approximately 180 mmHg unless the monitor identifies that you need a higher value. The cuff will then deflate automatically, and the numbers on the display screen will begin to drop. When the heart symbol stops flashing, your blood pressure and pulse readings will be displayed.

Some models are a combination of manual and automatic. That is, they do not use a stethoscope and you must squeeze a bulb to inflate the cuff, which is attached to a display monitor.

In the beginning, regardless of which type of blood pressure device you use, you should take a total of three readings, waiting 5–10 minutes between each recording. Once you become comfortable with using the device, one or two readings should be sufficient.

What Will the Results Tell Me?

Taking your blood pressure at home can help you monitor the effectiveness of any efforts you are taking to manage hypertension, whether that includes medications, diet, and/or exercise. Home monitoring also allows you to know if and when you should see your doctor about elevated blood pressure levels. Briefly:

- < 120/< 80 is normal blood pressure

- 120–139/80–89 is prehypertension

- 140–159/90–99 is stage 1 hypertension

- 160+/100+ is stage 2 hypertension

If your blood pressure is normal, maintaining or adopting a healthy lifestyle (good nutrition, no smoking, regular exercise, stress management) can prevent or delay the onset of high blood pressure and other health problems. If your blood pressure is not normal, a healthy lifestyle, and possibly medication, especially in stage 2, can help control your pressure and reduce your risk of life-threatening conditions. If you also have diabetes, chronic kidney disease, heart disease, a history of stroke, or certain other conditions, you and your doctor will likely take a more aggressive approach to treatment.

CHOLESTEROL TEST
Why Do I Need This Test?
An elevated cholesterol level is one indicator of risk for coronary heart disease. For people who are concerned about their cholesterol level because of family

history of heart disease or who want to monitor their cholesterol level because they have heart disease, a home test kit can be helpful and is convenient.

Home cholesterol test kits have been available over the counter since 1993. They have been approved by the Food and Drug Administration (FDA) and, when used correctly, they are accurate up to 95 percent of the time.

How Do I Use This Test?

It is important to remember to fast when taking a home cholesterol test because if you don't your results will likely be much higher than they actually are. Forgetting to fast is one of the most common mistakes people make when using this test.

The test kits typically include a test device, a cholesterol result chart, one or more lancets, gauze pad, bandage, and instructions. Just one or two drops of blood from your fingertip are typically needed for analysis. After 10–15 minutes, depending on the kit, you will read the test device, which is similar to a thermometer, to get your cholesterol reading. You should use the cholesterol conversion chart that comes with the kit to interpret your test results. Each chart is calibrated to each lot of test kits during the manufacturing process.

What Will the Results Tell Me?

Many home cholesterol tests give you a total cholesterol level only. That means you do not have information on LDL (low-density lipoprotein; or "bad" cholesterol) and HDL (high-density lipoprotein; or "good" cholesterol) levels. You need these figures to get an accurate picture of the state of your cholesterol. Some newer tests, however, also give LDL, HDL, triglyceride, and/or glucose (sugar) readings. In any case, a home cholesterol test kit does not replace a clinical test, nor does it offer an overall assessment of other risk factors for cardiovascular disease. You should inform your physician of your test results.

COLORECTAL DISEASE TEST

Why Do I Need This Test?

In their early stages, colorectal diseases such as cancers, ulcers, hemorrhoids, polyps, colitis, diverticulitis, and fissures may not present any symptoms or show any visible sign of blood, even though they may be producing blood hidden in the stool. A colorectal home test can detect unseen blood and alert you to bowel problems that may require medical attention.

The American Cancer Society and the U.S. Centers for Disease Control and Prevention (CDC) recommend annual testing for colorectal disease for everyone older than 50. If you have a family history of colorectal cancer or intestinal bleeding, the test should be done at an earlier age, more often, or as your doctor recommends.

How Do I Use This Test?

Two days before you take this test, avoid taking aspirin or any medications that contain aspirin, anti-inflammatory drugs, and rectal ointments. If you are taking medications, including prescribed doses of iron, consult with your doctor before using this test. You do not need to restrict your diet before taking this test, although it is recommended that you try to eat vegetables, fruits, and cereals for two days before and during the testing period. Do not use the test if you are menstruating, if you have bleeding hemorrhoids, or if you have constipation.

To prepare for the test, carefully read the preparation instructions that come with the kit. Different test kits differ slightly in their routine. Generally, remove all toilet cleaners, disinfectants, or deodorizers from the toilet bowl and tank. Flush the toilet bowl several times before beginning the test.

Place the test pad into the toilet after you have a bowel movement. Wait two minutes to see if the pad changes color. Test kits typically contain 3 testing pads, so you can repeat the test 2 more times over the next few days.

What Will the Results Tell Me?

If there is any change in color in the test area of the test pad, this indicates that blood may be present in your stool (a positive test result), and you should consult your doctor for further testing. Remember, however, that a positive test result does not necessarily mean that you have a problem. Follow-up testing by your physician can make that determination.

If you have a negative test result (no color change in the test area of the pad), it indicates that at the time of the testing, there was no detectable blood in your stool. A negative result is not a guarantee that there are no problems in the bowel, as some conditions do not cause bleeding all the time. If your test result is negative but you still have the following signs and/or symptoms, consult your doctor: diarrhea or constipation that lasts longer than two weeks, unexplained weight loss, black and/or tarry stool, and visible blood in the stool.

DRUG (ILLICIT) TEST
Why Do I Need This Test?
Home tests for illicit drugs are typically done by parents or guardians who want to see if their children are using drugs. Warning signs and symptoms of drug abuse can include but are not limited to neglected appearance or hygiene, poor self-image, violent outbursts, unexplained weight loss, slurred speech, skin sores or abrasions, glassy or red eyes, stealing, depression, withdrawal, apathy, reckless behavior, chemical smell to the breath, frequent use of eyedrops, disrespect to parents, lying, sneaky behavior, verbal abuse, lack of motivation, truancy, and manipulative behavior.

Home drug tests can be used to check for use of the most common street drugs, including methamphetamines (speed, ecstasy), cocaine, opiates (morphine, heroin), THC (marijuana), and PCP. Tests are also available to check for alcohol use. This entry focuses on illicit drugs.

How Do I Use This Test?

There are three testing methods: saliva, urine, and hair testing, and several different manufacturers of each type of testing kit. Each method has its benefits and drawbacks. Test kits are available to detect anything from a single drug up to 10–12 drugs per kit. Here is a general explanation of each testing method. You will need to follow the specific instructions provided with the test kit you choose.

Urine testing is the approach most commonly used by parents, employers, and law enforcement. It is also the most inexpensive method. It can detect drugs in a person's system for up to three days after they have used the drug. In some cases a test can detect substances up to 30 days after use, but you should not rely on this extended amount of time. Generally, if you suspect drug use occurred within the past few days, a urine drug test is your best choice. It can test for a single drug or many, depending on which kit you choose.

Urine drug testing kits are easy to use: one or more test strips are dipped into a urine sample, and after a few minutes you will be able to read the marks on the strips that indicate whether one or more drugs is in the urine. You should be sure the individual supplying the urine sample does not have an opportunity to cheat or adulterate the sample by adding chemicals. If necessary, you may need to perform the test more than once. Practicing random drug testing is the best way to prevent cheating or adulteration of the samples.

Saliva testing is an ideal choice to use on the day you suspect drug abuse has occurred or up to 48 hours after. The test is simple to use: you place the spoon collector or swab into the mouth of the individual, take a saliva sample, and place the collection item into the testing device. Results are ready within minutes and are indicated by a change in color on the testing device or swab. A drawback of the test is that if the individual also smokes cigarettes or chews gum often, the test results may be inaccurate. In that case, you may need to repeat the test.

Hair testing is the most accurate consumer drug test method on the market, and they are not easy to adulterate. Bleach, shampoos, and diet will not affect the results, even though there are bleaches and shampoos designed to help people cheat on these tests. Hair testing has the advantage of allowing you to test for possible drug use for up to 90 days of suspected abuse. All you need is a 1-½-inch sample of hair, as each half inch represents 30 days of growth. Drawbacks include higher cost and having to send the sample to a laboratory for testing and waiting for the results.

What Will the Results Tell Me?

Results of urine and saliva tests are immediate and will let you know whether the drugs for which you tested are present in the urine or saliva. Test kits have cutoff levels for each drug, below which they cannot detect any given drug. Drug detection times in urine vary:

- Amphetamines and methamphetamines: 1–4 days

- Barbiturates: short-acting, 1–3 days; long-acting, 1–3 weeks

- Benzodiazepines: short-term use, 1–3 days; long-term use, 1–3 weeks

- Cocaine: 1–5 days

- Ecstasy: 1–4 days

- LSD: 1–2 days

- Marijuana: casual use, 1–7 days; long-term use, 1–4 weeks

- Methadone: 1–4 days

- Opiates: 1–5 days

- PCP: casual use, 1–7 days; long-term use, 1–4 weeks

Hair test results can tell you the amount of drug(s) in the person's system and what type of user the person is (e.g., low, medium, or high user). Hair testing will not detect drug use within the last seven days, as the hair needs time to grow. If you get a negative result and you still suspect drug use, you can use a saliva test.

In all cases, home drug test results are only preliminary. You should seek a more specific testing method to get a confirmed analytic result. The most typical testing method is gas chromatography-mass spectrometry, the approach preferred by the National Institute on Drug Abuse.

GLUCOSE (SUGAR) TESTING
Why Do I Need This Test?
Home blood sugar testing can be used to monitor your blood sugar levels at your convenience. People who have diabetes usually need to check their levels at least once a day, and those who require insulin to control their diabetes may need to check their sugar levels several times daily.

It's important to know when your blood sugar is high (hyperglycemia) or low (hypoglycemia) to prevent glucose or insulin reactions. Blood sugar levels that are consistently high need to be treated to decrease your chances of developing heart, blood vessel, and nerve complications associated with diabetes.

Testing your blood sugar levels can help you decide how much insulin you need to take before each meal, how to better schedule your insulin, and how exercise, diet, stress, and being ill is affecting your blood sugar levels.

How Do I Use This Test?

To test your blood sugar, you need a blood glucose meter, testing strips, lancets for pricking your skin, a lancet holder, rubbing alcohol, and clean cotton balls.

Always check the expiration date on your testing strips, because expired ones will not give you an accurate reading. Because each glucose meter is different, you should make sure you understand how to use the meter. Your doctor, nurse, or pharmacist can help you if you have any questions.

To use a home blood sugar test, you need to do the following:

- Clean your finger or other site from which you will be getting the blood sample. You can use alcohol on a cotton ball or cotton-swab.

- Insert a clean lancet into the lancet holder.

- Remove a test strip from the bottle. Some testing strips are stored inside the meter.

- Prick your finger or other site.

- Put the drop of blood on the correct spot on the test strip.

- Use a clean cotton ball to apply pressure where you pricked your finger or other site.

- Follow the directions with your meter to get your results. Some meters provide results immediately.

- Record your results. Most meters will store results for weeks so you can retrieve them later.

What Will the Results Tell Me?

Normal results before meals are 70–130 milligrams per deciliter (mg/dL); after meals, less than 180 mg/dL. Values can vary depending on your activity level, your food intake, and your use of insulin. Low glucose levels indicate hypoglycemia, and you should have something to eat. It may also indicate a need to change your next dose of insulin. If your results are too high, this indicates hyperglycemia. If you use insulin, you may need to take more. Consult your doctor about the meaning of your specific test results.

Some glucose meters can store hundreds of glucose readings, which allows you to spot any major changes in your sugar levels and also to predict levels at certain times of the day. Certain models also allow information to be downloaded to a computer. Some newer models of home glucose meters can communicate with insulin pumps, which can help you determine how much insulin you need.

HEMOGLOBIN A1C
Why Do I Need This Test?
The hemoglobin A1c test (HbA1c) reveals the rate that blood sugar binds to the hemoglobin molecules in red blood cells and provides an indication of average blood sugar control. It is especially important for people who have diabetes, as it tells them how they have managed their disease over the last 90 days. Why 90 days? Because that's the average life of red blood cells. If a person with diabetes has a high HbA1c reading, it indicates that there needs to be a change in how they are controlling their sugar levels.

Adequate control of blood sugar levels is important because high levels greatly increase the risk of developing damaging and life-threatening complications, such as neuropathy, blindness, impotence, stroke, heart attack, and amputation.

The American Diabetes Association recommends that people with diabetes test both their blood glucose and their HbA1c.

How Do I Take This Test?
The test kit contains instructions, lancet, test form, and the prepaid mailing supplies. To take the test, wash your hands, and then stick your finger with the lancet. Place two drops of blood on the test strip on the test form. Allow the blood to dry overnight and then mail it to the laboratory.

To avoid an extra finger stick, you can collect your test sample at the same time you are testing your blood glucose levels.

What Will the Results Tell Me?

Results are usually available within 7–8 business days. They will be mailed to you.

In people who do not have diabetes, the normal A1c range is 4 to 6 percent. People with diabetes typically have levels around 8–9 percent, but research, as well as the American Diabetes Association, recommends levels below 7 as ideal. That's because every 1 percent increase above 6 percent raises the risk of diabetes-related problems. Thus an A1c that is 8 percent or higher is a sign that patients should consult their health-care provider to change their treatment plan. A level of 7 percent or lower is an indication that the current treatment plan is working and that blood sugar levels are under control.

HEPATITIS C TEST

Why Do I Need This Test?

A home hepatitis C test allows you to test for this serious disease in the privacy of your home or office. Hepatitis C usually has no symptoms in the early stages, and people can carry the virus for up to 20 years before learning that they have the disease. Hepatitis C is the tenth leading cause of death in the United States. An estimated 3.9 million Americans are infected, and about 8,000–10,000 people die annually from chronic liver disease that is caused by the virus. Early detection of hepatitis C allows you to begin treatment to avoid more serious conditions, including cirrhosis and liver cancer.

How Do I Use This Test?

Currently there is only one FDA-approved hepatitis C home test kit on the market. The test kit was developed for screening and identifying the human hepatitis C virus in whole blood. The test comes with a small blotter, which is identified with a unique 14-digit number, and a device that allows you to prick your finger. Before you take the test, you are advised to call the toll-free number that comes with the kit and register your PIN (personal identification number). This allows your results to remain anonymous. After you prick your finger, you place a few drops of blood on the blotter and ship it in the prepaid mailer to the lab indicated.

What Will the Results Tell Me?

Use of this test provides you with anonymity and privacy. The results are available in about 10 business days. You may call a toll-free number anonymously and access your test results using your unique 14-digit code or get your results in the mail. If you test positive for hepatitis C, you should contact your physician. If you do not have a physician and/or you want to discuss the results, you can talk with counselors associated with the home test provider by calling the same toll-free number and asking for physician referral and/or further information.

HIV TESTING
Why Do I Need This Test?

Details about HIV testing are discussed in the "25 Common Medical Tests" section of this book. The specific advantage of a home HIV test is privacy: when you mail in your test sample, you are identified only by a code number that comes with the kit. You also have access to anonymous phone support from the testing service.

How Do I Use This Test?

Use an FDA-approved test kit only. HIV home test kits can be purchased online, by fax or mail order, or through retail pharmacies. The kits come with detailed instructions that take you through pretest registration and counseling, how to collect the blood sample, how to ship the sample to the laboratory, and when to call for test results, post-test counseling, and referrals.

The first step is to call the toll-free number to register your anonymous code number and complete pretest counseling. This can be accomplished with a counselor over the phone or through an automated registration and education system.

To collect the blood sample, use the retractable lancet in the kit, prick your finger, and place drops of blood on the provided specimen card. Place the sample in the weather-resistant pouch that comes with the kit and place it in the self-addressed, prepaid shipping envelope.

What Will the Results Tell Me?

It typically takes about seven days after you send your sample for your results to become available. You can get your results by calling the toll-free number and giving the counselor your special code number. You also have access to a counselor who can talk to you about your results and your options. See "What Will the Results Tell Me?" under the "HIV Testing" section in Chapter 2 of this book.

LEAD TESTING

Why Do I Need This Test?

This test can help you ensure that you and your family have not been exposed to dangerous levels of lead. You may want to use this test if you are in an environment that had lead-based paint (e.g., an older home or building), especially if it is peeling. Lead exposure can also come from drinking water, contaminated soil, defective glazes on pottery, and in airborne particulates. In recent years, lead has been found on children's toys that have been imported from China.

Although people of any age can suffer from lead poisoning, children are affected much more frequently. Approximately 310,000 children between the ages of 1 and 5 years in the United States have blood levels of lead greater than 10 micrograms per deciliter of blood (mcg/dL). At that level, the Centers for Disease Control and Prevention recommends that parents identify and reduce exposure to help prevent the damage that high levels can do. Exposure to lead and lead dust can interfere with some of the body's basic functions. Because the body cannot differentiate between lead and calcium, it absorbs both into the bones, where it can accumulate throughout a person's life. Even low exposure to lead can affect children and result in anemia, colic, poor muscle coordination, hearing damage, speech and language problems, kidney damage, learning disabilities, reduced muscle and bone growth, and impaired vitamin D metabolism.

How Do I Use This Test?

There are several lead test kits on the market. All of them involve the use of disposable swabs that change color to indicate the presence of lead and, in some cases, other metals such as barium and/or tin. Different test brands utilize different colors. Typically, the swabs are either self-contained and have been treated with either rhodizonate ion or sulfide ion (both of which are nontoxic and odorless), or you must dip them into a vial that contains one of these chemicals before you apply the swab to the test surface to detect lead. The swabs can be applied to just about any surface, including vinyl, fabric, rugs, walls, metal, and plastic. In some cases the swab will change color within seconds, indicating the presence of lead. If there are very low levels of lead, it may take an hour or more for the swab to change color.

What Will the Results Tell Me?

In 2007, the U.S. Consumer Product Safety Commission (CPSC) reported on the results of their evaluation of consumer lead test kits and found that slightly more than half of the 104 test results they gathered were false negatives and two were false positives. None of the test kits they evaluated consistently detected lead in products if the items were covered with a nonleaded coating.

Consumers should check with the CPSC and/or *Consumer Reports* before purchasing a home lead test kit to learn which ones are the most reliable. Items that test positive should be removed from use. Home test kits can detect surface but not embedded lead. To get exact lead levels, you will need to hire a professional.

MICROALBUMIN TEST

Why Do I Need This Test?

This test measures the levels of a protein called albumin. Albumin is normally found in the blood and filtered by the kidneys. When the kidneys are functioning properly, there is no albumin in the urine. When the kidneys are damaged, however, albumin leaks into the urine. This condition is called microalbuminuria. Early detection of microalbumin in urine is important to help prevent kidney disease, a major complication of diabetes.

The American Diabetes Association (ADA) and the American Kidney Foundation recommend that everyone with diabetes be tested for microalbuminuria annually. According to the ADA, 20–30 percent of people who have diabetes develop kidney disease. However, microalbuminuria can be caused by other factors as well, such as high blood pressure, heart failure, cirrhosis, or systemic lupus erythematosus.

If kidney damage is not caught early and treated, larger amounts of albumin can get into the urine. This condition is called macroalbuminuria or proteinuria. This often indicates serious kidney damage and can lead to chronic kidney disease.

How Do I Take the Test?

Not all microalbumin test kits are the same. One type requires you to send a liquid urine sample; another type lets you send a dried urine sample on a paddle. Regardless of the type of test, however, you must collect a clean-catch midstream urine sample. A morning urine sample provides the best information about albumin levels.

Before collecting the urine sample, men should first clean the head of the penis with medicated swabs or towelettes. Women should spread open the folds of skin around the vagina with one hand and use the other hand to clean the vaginal and urethra area thoroughly with medicated swabs or towelettes. Begin urinating into the toilet or urinal. After the urine has flowed for several seconds, place the collection cup into the stream and collect about 2 ounces. Do not touch the rim of the cup to the genital area or get any foreign matter (e.g., menstrual blood, feces, pubic hair) into the sample.

What Will the Results Tell Me?

A normal albumin reading is less than 30 mg of albumin in 24 hours. You should consult your doctor if your results are higher. Levels between 165 and 300 mg of albumin in 24 hours indicates microalbuminuria and that you should have your urine checked regularly to watch for kidney damage. Levels of 300 mg or higher is macroalbuminuria.

Your test results may not be useful if you have high blood sugar levels, a urinary tract infection, high blood pressure, heart failure, or high fever. Use of medication such as aspirin, corticosteroids, and some antibiotics can affect the results. Having menstrual bleeding or vaginal discharge may temporarily affect a urine sample.

OVULATION TEST
Why Do I Need This Test?

For women who are trying to get pregnant, this test can tell them when they are ovulating and help them plan their pregnancy. The test detects a hormone called luteinizing hormone (LH), which is always present in the body in small amounts. Levels of the hormone rise significantly, however, around the middle of the menstrual cycle, when the pituitary gland releases it in greater quantities than any other time during the cycle. The increase lasts for up to three days, and this is the time when women are most likely to ovulate and thus most able to become pregnant.

How Do I Take the Test?

The home ovulation tests use urine. You will collect a urine sample in a small container and then dip the test strip into the sample. It is recommended that you reduce your intake of liquids for 2 hours before taking the test.

To decide when to begin testing, determine the length of your normal menstrual cycle. The length of a cycle is from the beginning of one period to the beginning of the next. The beginning is defined as the first day of bleeding or spotting. If your menstrual cycle varies by more than a few days each month, take the average number of days for the last 3 months. The kit contains a chart that can help you determine the day you should begin testing.

What Will the Results Tell Me?

The results of the test appear on a test strip: one line tells you the test is working, while the appearance of a second line that is the same or a darker color than the first indicates that you should ovulate soon. The surge in LH normally occurs 12–36 hours after ovulation, and women are most likely to become pregnant if they have intercourse within 36 hours after detecting the surge.

PREGNANCY TEST

Why Do I Need This Test?

A home pregnancy test allows you to discover whether you are pregnant in the privacy of your home and at your convenience. Home pregnancy tests measure the presence of a hormone called human chorionic gonadotropin (hCG) in the urine, which is an indicator of pregnancy. Human chorionic gonadotropin, which is produced by cells from the placenta, first enters the bloodstream when the fertilized egg implants in the uterus, which is about 6 days after fertilization. The level of hCG then increases rapidly, doubling about every 2 days.

How Do I Take the Test?

Although there are various types of home pregnancy tests, most work in a similar way. You will place the end of a dipstick in your urine stream or immerse the dipstick in a container into which you have collected a urine sample. After a minute or two, the dipstick will reveal a plus or minus sign, a color change, a line, or the words "pregnant" or "not pregnant." A few tests involve mixing a small amount of urine with a special liquid or powder. If the urine changes color, the test is positive.

Because instructions may vary slightly from test to test, be sure to read the directions carefully, especially if you are doing a retest and are using a different test kit. If you have any questions about the kit, how to do the test, or how to interpret your results, contact the manufacturer, whose toll-free number and/or Web site information should be on the package. Here are some other tips on using a home pregnancy test kit:

• For best results, you should test first thing in the morning, when your urine is most concentrated. However, if this is not possible, make sure the urine you use has been in your bladder for at least 4 hours.

• To help ensure you read your test correctly, have a watch or clock nearby so you can time the length of the test accurately. If you read the test too early or too late, you may skew the results.

• If you are taking any type of medication (e.g., fertility drugs), read the package inserts before you take the test to see if the medications will affect the results.

• Do not drink an excessive amount of water before the test in an attempt to increase the volume of urine, because this can dilute the concentration of hCG and give you an inaccurate result.

What Will the Results Tell Me?

Some home pregnancy tests claim to allow you to learn whether you are pregnant as early as 7 days after conception or that you can use them as early as the day you miss your period. However, research shows that this claim is misleading. Although some tests may detect hCG in urine at this point and give a positive result, most are not sensitive enough to guarantee that the result is accurate. Experts recommend, therefore, that women wait one week after their expected period before taking a home pregnancy test.

You may get a negative result for several reasons. You may not be pregnant, you may have taken the test too early, you may have ovulated later than you thought (therefore there's not enough hCG to detect yet), or you are pregnant but you have complications that affect the amount of hCG in your body. If you get a negative result, experts recommend you test again after a few days if you still have not gotten your period.

If your test is positive, or if you have taken several home pregnancy tests and you have gotten mixed results, contact your doctor, nurse practitioner, or midwife. You may need to take a blood test or have a pelvic examination to confirm that you are pregnant. If your test results are still negative two weeks after you have missed your period, call your doctor. You may be missing your period for a variety of reasons, including stress, hormonal imbalance, or illness.

VAGINAL PH (YEAST INFECTION) TEST
Why Do I Need This Test?
For many women, the first thing that comes to mind when they experience unusual vaginal symptoms

(e.g., foul vaginal odor, itching, burning, abnormal vaginal discharge) is "Do I have a yeast infection?" In many cases, the answer is yes. About 75 percent of women have at least one yeast infection during their lives, nearly 50 percent have two or more, and 5 percent experience four or more.

Vaginal yeast infections are caused by an overgrowth of the fungus *Candida albicans*. Because the signs and symptoms of a yeast infections are very similar to those of sexually transmitted diseases, which can lead to serious consequences if not treated promptly, it is important that you make sure you have a yeast infection and not something more serious. Correctly identifying a yeast infection before treating it is important because use of antifungal medications when you don't really have a yeast infection can increase your risk of getting a difficult-to-treat infection in the future.

How Do I Use This Test?

The home vaginal pH test typically includes a piece of pH test paper or a cotton swab and a color chart that helps you determine your test results. To do the test, hold the pH test paper against the wall of your vagina for a few seconds, or swipe the cotton swab inside your vagina. Then, compare the color of your pH test paper or swab to the colors on the chart. Choose the color that most closely matches the one on your test paper.

Another type of vaginal pH test involves wearing a specially treated panty liner, which collects vaginal secretions. Like the pH test or cotton swab, you compare the color of the panty liner against a color chart.

Read the instructions carefully. Generally, vaginal pH tests should be used only by women who have normal menstrual periods. The test should not be used for 72 hours after you have used any type of vaginal preparation, such as contraceptive creams or products to treat internal yeast infection. You also should not use the test within 48 hours of sexual intercourse or douching or within 5 days of menses. Perimenopause, menopause, or the presence of blood, semen, or cervical mucus can cause abnormal vaginal pH results.

What Do the Results Tell Me?

A home vaginal pH test kit measures pH on a scale of 1 to 14. Normal vaginal pH is 3.8 to 4.5, which is slightly acidic. An abnormal reading is one that is higher or lower than the normal range. Although an abnormal vaginal pH frequently indicates the presence of a vaginal infection, not all vaginal infections cause the vaginal pH to change. In other words, just because your test results come out normal does not mean you do not have a vaginal infection.

If your vaginal pH value is above normal, the most likely reason is that you have bacterial vaginosis, which is not a yeast infection. You will need to see your doctor to get a definitive diagnosis and treatment. If your vaginal pH is within normal range or below normal and you are still experiencing symptoms, it is likely (but not definite) that you have a vaginal yeast infection. In such cases, you may want to use one of the over-the-counter yeast infection medications, especially if you have had a yeast infection in the past that has responded to such treatment. If, however, the over-the-counter medication does not cure your symptoms, you should contact your doctor for a definitive diagnosis and treatment.

It is important to note that a home vaginal pH test will not diagnose human immunodeficiency virus (HIV), chlamydia, herpes, gonorrhea, syphilis, or group B streptococcus. Therefore, if home treatment does not work, you should see your physician or go to a local clinic as soon as possible to get tested for sexually transmitted diseases.

VITAMIN D DEFICIENCY TEST
Why Do I Need This Test?
Vitamin D deficiency is common, and can be found in people of all ages. Although experts do not agree completely on how prevalent vitamin D deficiency is, generally it appears to impact about 40 percent of the overall population, with certain populations having much greater deficits. For example, about 60 percent of hospitalized individuals, 80 percent of people in nursing homes, and 48 percent of girls ages 9–11 have a vitamin D deficiency. Severe vitamin D deficiency is seen among pregnant women, which can lead to widespread deficiencies in their unborn children. Therefore, even if you do not fall into one of

the special categories, there's a good chance you have a vitamin D deficiency.

Abnormally low levels of vitamin D carry a potential for various health problems. Research shows that low vitamin D levels can contribute to the risk of breast cancer, heart disease, colon cancer, osteoporosis, multiple sclerosis, insomnia, fibromyalgia and other autoimmune diseases, and depression.

How Do I Use This Test?

A home vitamin D test involves taking a blood sample from your finger or heel and placing a few drops of blood on a special blotting paper that is included in the kit. The kit contains the blotting paper, a lancet for you to take the blood sample, a container for the blood sample, and a prepaid envelope for you to mail the sample to the laboratory.

What Will the Results Tell Me?

If your vitamin D level is below 20 ng/mL (nanograms per milliliter), this indicates a deficiency. Levels between 20 and 30 ng/mL are considered low, while levels greater than 150 ng/mL are toxic. The average person starts to store vitamin D (cholecalciferol) at 40 ng/mL, but when the body takes in 50 ng/mL, virtually everyone begins to store the vitamin for future use. According to the Vitamin D Council, the optimal levels of vitamin D in the body should be between 50 and 80 ng/mL.

If your test results indicate that you have a vitamin D deficiency or that your levels are low, you should talk to your doctor about how to supplement properly. It is possible to overdose on vitamin D, but only with supplements. Exposure to the sun, which allows the body to produce the vitamin, will not result in an overdose because once the body's requirements have been met, vitamin production stops until the need arises again. You also cannot overdose on food sources of vitamin D (except cod liver oil). Taking high doses of vitamin D supplements, however, can cause hypervitaminosis D. This can occur because vitamin D is a fat-soluble vitamin and it can accumulate in the fat cells of the body to toxic levels. Hypervitaminosis D is characterized by abnormally high levels of calcium in the blood. Symptoms include constipation, decreased appetite, dehydration, vomiting, fatigue, and irritability. Left untreated, hypervitaminosis D can eventually damage the bones, kidneys, and soft tissues.

CHAPTER 4

CONDITIONS AND DISEASES

So now you've reached the last chapter, where we talk about diseases and health conditions. Why did we include this chapter, and how did we go about selecting the entries that are in it?

The information in this chapter may help you better understand why your health-care provider ordered a specific diagnostic or screening test, gain more information about a condition you may have already been diagnosed with, and/or which tests are more commonly ordered or recommended for that condition. Each entry begins with the test or tests that are usually recommended and that have been covered in this book. In some cases, these tests are followed by one or more tests that doctors use, but which we do not discuss in this volume.

The information in this chapter may prompt you to ask your doctor about his or her choice of tests and/or pique your interest to learn more on your own about a specific medical condition and the tests used to diagnose it. It may also make you think about trying a home test kit—or at least investigating them further.

The bottom line is that the more information you have as a health-care consumer, the better equipped and confident you can be when you meet with your doctor or other health-care practitioner to talk about your symptoms, tests, and test results.

The medical conditions and disorders in this chapter were chosen because they affect a large number of people both directly and indirectly. The entry on asthma, for example, notes that more than 22 million people in the United States suffer from this condition. There are about 182,000 new cases of breast cancer diagnosed each year, and 13 million people have coronary artery disease. Accordingly, some of the most common medical diagnostic and screening tests on the market are typically ordered or recommended to identify or diagnose these conditions. Thus, the information in this chapter complements what we have provided in chapters 2 and 3.

Naturally, we could not hope to discuss each of the medical conditions and diseases in depth. That's why we invite you to check out the Appendix at the end of the book for sources of additional information from knowledgeable and reliable literature, organizations, and Web sites.

ABDOMINAL AORTIC ANEURYSM

Tests that help diagnose or screen for this condition: an abdominal ultrasound is the best diagnostic test.

An abdominal aortic aneurysm is an abnormal bulge or ballooning of the wall of the aorta in the abdomen. The aorta is a major blood vessel that provides blood to the body. Because it is the body's main supplier of blood, a ruptured aortic aneurysm can cause life-threatening bleeding. Although most small and slow-growing aortic aneurysms don't rupture, large, fast-growing ones may.

Abdominal aortic aneurysms are most often seen in men age 40–70. Possible causes of an abdominal aortic aneurysm include tobacco use (which contributes to atherosclerosis and high blood pressure, causing aneurysms to grow faster), high blood pressure (especially if not controlled well), and infection of the aorta (vasculitis).

Complications of an abdominal aortic aneurysm include rupture and blood clots. Blood clots can cause pain or restrict blood flow to the legs, toes, or abdominal organs.

Signs and symptoms: pain in the chest, abdomen, or lower back, possibly spreading to the groin, buttocks, or legs that may last for hours or days; pulsating sensation in the abdomen, back pain (if the aneurysm is pressing on the spine), fever or weight loss (if an inflammatory aortic aneurysm). Signs and symptoms that the aneurysm has burst include sudden intense and persistent abdominal pain, pain that radiates to the back or legs, sweatiness, dizziness, low blood pressure, fast pulse, loss of consciousness, and shortness of breath.

ASTHMA

Tests that help diagnose or screen for this condition: pulmonary function tests.

Asthma is a chronic lung disease characterized by inflammation and narrowing of the airways. It can affect people of any age, but it most often first appears in childhood. More than 22 million people in the United States have asthma, and nearly 6 million of these are children.

People with asthma have inflamed bronchi, which are tubes that transport air into and out of the lungs. The inflammation makes the airways very sensitive, so they can react strongly to certain substances when they are inhaled. When the airways react, the muscles around them tighten, causing the airways to narrow and the airflow to be significantly reduced. The cells in the bronchi may also produce more mucus than normal, which can further narrow the airways. This chain reaction of events can occur every time the airways are irritated.

Signs and symptoms: coughing (often worse at night or early in the morning), wheezing, chest tightness, shortness of breath.

BENIGN PROSTATIC HYPERPLASIA

Tests that help diagnose or screen for this condition: prostate-specific antigen (PSA) test; also digital rectal examination, cystoscopy.

Benign prostatic hyperplasia (BPH), also known as benign prostatic hypertrophy, is a noncancerous (benign) condition in which the prostate gland becomes enlarged (hyperplasia). It is a very common condition, affecting more than half of all men age 50 and older. An enlarged prostate does not always cause symptoms, and only about 10 percent of men require medical or surgical treatment.

The exact cause of BPH is not known. One theory is that changes in the ratio of testosterone and estrogen levels may stimulate growth of the prostate. Aging is also believed to be a factor, as the prostate gland becomes more sensitive to normal levels of testosterone and grows faster.

An enlarged prostate can become a serious problem if it interferes with the ability to empty the bladder. Men who have BPH are at increased risk of urinary tract infections, development of bladder stones, kidney damage, bladder damage, and acute urinary retention, which is a sudden painful inability to urinate.

Signs and symptoms: need to urinate frequently, slow flow of urine, urgent need to urinate, difficulty starting urination, urinary tract infections, pain in the pelvic region.

BREAST CANCER

Tests that help diagnose or screen for this condition: clinical breast examination, mammogram (screening and/or diagnostic); also breast self-examination.

Breast cancer is cancer that forms in tissues of the breast, usually in the ducts and lobules (glands that produce milk). Although it occurs in both women and men, it is rare in men. According to the National Cancer Institute, in 2008, more than 182,000 new cases were diagnosed in women and 1,990 in men. Most cases of breast cancer in women occur after menopause and in women age 60 or older.

In most cases it is not known what causes normal breast cells to become cancerous. Only 5–10 percent of breast cancers are inherited, caused by genetic defects in one of two genes, breast cancer gene 1 or gene 2 (BRCA1, BRCA2). There are also other in-herited mutations that make it more likely to develop breast cancer.

There are two main types of breast cancer: in situ and invasive. In situ (noninvasive) breast cancer re-fers to cancer in which the cells do not spread to breast tissue around the duct or lobule. The most common type of noninvasive breast cancer is ductal carcinoma in situ, which is located in the lining of the milk ducts. Invasive breast cancers spread out-side the membrane that lines a lobule or duct, and the cells can then travel to other parts of the body. About 70 percent of all breast cancers are invasive ductal carcinoma, in which the cancer cells first form in the lining of the milk duct and then break through the wall and invade other breast tissue. The cancer cells may then remain in that location or spread (metastasize) throughout the body.

Signs and symptoms: a lump or thickening in or near the breast or under the arm; nipple tenderness; a change in the size or shape of the breast; a nipple that turns inward into the breast; skin of the breast, areola, or nipple becomes scaly, red, swollen, or has ridges or pitting that looks like the skin of an orange; discharge from the nipple.

BRONCHITIS
Tests that help diagnose or screen for this condition: pulmonary function tests; also chest X-rays.

Bronchitis is an acute inflammation of the airways within the lungs. It occurs when the windpipe (trachea) and the large and small airways (bronchi) become inflamed due to an upper respiratory infection such as the common cold or a sinus infection. Most cases of acute bronchitis resolve within a few days, although coughs may linger for a few weeks. Cases of bronchitis that keep recurring may develop into chronic bronchitis, which can lead to asthma or other serious conditions.

People of any age can get bronchitis. Infants usually get bronchiolitis, which affects the smaller airways and causes symptoms that are similar to asthma.

Signs and symptoms: cough (may be dry or produce phlegm), wheezing; also may have fever with chills, muscle aches, nasal congestion, sore throat.

CERVICAL CANCER
Tests that help diagnose or screen for this condition: Pap smear.

Cervical cancer is a cancer that forms in the tissues of the cervix. It is typically a slow-growing cancer that often does not present with symptoms. There are two main types of cervical cancers: squamous cell carcinoma and adenocarcinoma. Between 80 and 90 percent of cervical cancers are squamous cell carcinomas, which arise from cells that cover the surface of the exocervix (the part of the cervix closest to the body of the uterus). Most of the remaining 10–20 percent are adenocarcinomas, which develops from the mucus-producing gland cells of the endocervix. Adenocarcinomas are becoming more common in women born in the 1980s and 1990s. Rarely cervical cancers have features of both squamous cell carcinomas and adenocarcinomas.

According to the National Cancer Institute, an estimated 11,070 new cases of cervical cancer were diagnosed in the United States in 2008.

Signs and symptoms: Women often do not notice symptoms because they mimic so many other conditions, including premenstrual syndrome and ovulation pain. When symptoms are present, they usually appear when the cancer is more advanced. When symptoms do occur, they may include abnormal vaginal bleeding, unusual heavy vaginal discharge (may be watery, thick, foul-smelling, or contain mucus), pelvic pain, pain during urination, bleeding between regular menstrual periods and/or after sexual intercourse.

CHRONIC OBSTRUCTIVE PULMONARY DISEASE

Tests that help diagnose or screen for this condition: pulmonary function tests; also chest X-rays, sputum analysis.

Chronic obstructive pulmonary disease (COPD) is a general term for a progressive disease that makes it difficult to breathe. The two main COPD conditions are emphysema and chronic obstructive bronchitis. In emphysema, the walls between the air sacs in the lungs are damaged, which can cause the sacs to lose their shape and become less effective. Some air sacs may also be destroyed. In chronic obstructive bronchitis, the lining of the airways is always inflamed and irritated, which leads to a thickening of the lining and thus difficulty breathing.

Most people who have COPD have both emphysema and chronic obstructive bronchitis. More than 12 million people in the United States have been diagnosed with COPD, and another 12 million probably have the disease and don't know it. The leading cause of COPD is cigarette smoking; long-term exposure to air pollutants, dust, or chemical fumes may contribute to the disease. It is usually diagnosed in middle-aged or older people.

Signs and symptoms: Symptoms develop slowly over time. Early symptoms and warning signs differ from person to person and can even be different between episodes in the same person. Signs and symptoms may include an increase or decrease in the amount of sputum produced, a change in color of sputum, presence of blood in sputum, increase in stickiness or thickness of sputum, increase in severity of shortness of breath, increase in severity of cough and/or wheezing, ankle swelling, forgetfulness, confusion, slurred speech, sleepiness, sleep difficulties, increased fatigue, lack of sex drive, increasing morning headaches, dizziness, and restlessness.

CIRRHOSIS

Tests that help diagnose or screen for this condition: liver function panel, complete blood count; also liver biopsy.

Cirrhosis is a term that describes scarring of the liver. When the damage to the liver is minor or mild, the liver can usually repair itself and continue its vital functions, which include detoxifying harmful substances in the body, purifying the blood, and producing essential nutrients. If, however, the damage is advanced or severe, more and more scar tissue forms, making it impossible for the liver to function and liver failure occurs.

Cirrhosis and chronic liver failure are leading causes of morbidity and death in the United States. Most of the cases are preventable, as they are associated with excessive alcohol consumption, viral hepatitis, or nonalcoholic fatty liver disease (related to diet). Most patients who have cirrhosis do not experience any noticeable symptoms until the disease is advanced.

Signs and symptoms: Cirrhosis usually does not have any signs or symptoms until the disease is advanced. When signs and symptoms do appear, they may include fatigue, bleeding easily, bruising easily, accumulation of fluid in the abdomen, loss of appetite, nausea, swelling in the legs, and weight loss.

COLORECTAL CANCER
Tests that help diagnose or screen for this condition: fecal occult blood, colonoscopy, barium enema; also flexible sigmoidoscopy.

Colorectal cancer is a term used to refer to cancer that originates in either the colon (large intestine) or the rectum (last 6 inches of the colon). According to the American Cancer Society, about 112,000 people are diagnosed with colon cancer each year, and about 41,000 new cases of rectal cancer are discovered annually.

Although cancer that starts in these different

areas of the intestinal tract may cause different symptoms (see below), they have many things in common. Generally, colorectal cancers develop gradually over many years and usually begin as a growth of noncancerous (benign) tissue called a polyp. A polyp may become cancerous over time, and removing it early may prevent it from becoming cancer. Thus early detection of polyps is critical.

More than 95 percent of colorectal cancers are adenocarcinomas, which are cancers that start in the cells that line the inside of the colon and rectum. Most colorectal cancers are diagnosed in people older than 50, but it can appear in people of any age. Risk factors include chronic ulcerative colitis, Crohn's disease, inflammatory bowel disease, intestinal polyps, and a diet high in fat.

Signs and symptoms: Many people with colorectal cancer do not experience symptoms in the early stages of the disease. When symptoms do occur, they can include changes in bowel habits, blood in the feces, rectal bleeding, feeling that your bowel will not empty completely, weakness, fatigue, unexplained weight loss, persistent cramping, gas, abdominal pain.

CORONARY ARTERY DISEASE
Tests that help diagnose or screen for this condition: complete blood count (CBC), electrocardiogram (EKG), exercise stress test; also echocardiogram.

Coronary artery disease (CAD), also called coronary heart disease, is condition in which plaque (fat, cholesterol, calcium, and other substances) accumulates inside the coronary arteries. It is the most common type of heart disease: it affects 13 million people in the United States and is the number one killer of adults in the nation. The buildup of plaque is called atherosclerosis, and it blocks the flow of oxygen-rich blood to the heart. Partially blocked arteries can cause chest pain or discomfort, called angina. When the blood flow to an area of the heart is completely blocked, a heart attack occurs. Over time, CAD causes the heart muscles to weaken, leading to heart failure and arrhythmia.

Signs and symptoms: chest pain (angina); pain in the abdomen, back, or arm (especially in women); shortness of breath; heart attack (symptoms include crushing pressure in chest and pain in shoulder or arm, shortness of breath, sweating; women are more likely to experience nausea and back or jaw pain).

DIABETES (TYPE 2)
Tests that help diagnose or screen for this condition: fasting blood glucose test; also glucose tolerance test.

Type 2 diabetes is the most common form of diabetes. Unlike type 1 diabetes, which is an autoimmune disorder that first appears in childhood, type 2 diabetes typically first manifests in adulthood and is largely associated with diet. In type 1 diabetes, the pancreas does not produce insulin; in type 2 diabetes, the body does not produce enough insulin or the body's cells do not respond appropriately to the insulin that is produced. The latest figures indicate that there are 23.6 million people with diabetes in the United States, and 90–95 percent of them have type 2.

The body needs insulin to be able to use glucose (sugar) for energy. After the body breaks down the food you consume into glucose, it is the job of insulin to take the glucose from the blood and into the cells. When insulin does not or cannot do its job, glucose accumulates in the blood instead of entering the cells. This causes two major problems: your body doesn't have enough energy, and over time, high levels of sugar in the blood can damage your kidneys, nerves, heart, and eyes.

Type 2 diabetes can occur in people of all races, although it is more common in African Americans, Latinos, Native Americans, and Asian Americans than in Caucasians. Although type 2 diabetes was once referred to as "adult-onset" diabetes because it was seen almost exclusively in adults, it is appearing in children and adolescents in rising numbers.

Signs and symptoms: Symptoms may not appear for years after diabetes develops. When they do occur they may include increased thirst, frequent urination, extreme hunger, weight loss, fatigue, irritability, blurry vision, and infections that are slow to heal. Vaginal and bladder infections are common in women. In some cases, patches of velvety dark skin may develop in the folds and creases of the body (e.g., neck, armpits). This is called acanthosis nigricans and is a sign of insulin resistance.

DIVERTICULOSIS/DIVERTICULITIS
Tests that help diagnose or screen for this condition: abdominal ultrasound; also computed tomography (CT)

These are two gastrointestinal disorders that affect the diverticula—the pouches in the lining of the colon (large intestine). When the diverticula bulge outward through weak spots in the intestine, the condition is called diverticulosis. If these pouches become inflamed, the condition is called diverticulitis. About 10 percent of Americans older than 40 have diverticulosis, with the prevalence increasing to about 50 percent among people older than 60. Approximately 10–25 percent of people who have diverticulosis develop diverticulitis. Together diverticulosis and diverticulitis are known as diverticular disease.

Diverticulitis can lead to infections, bleeding, perforation in the colon, and blockages in the colon. All of these complications require treatment to prevent more serious illness.

The cause of diverticular disease is not known.

However, the most popular theory is that a low-fiber diet, the diet practiced by most Americans, is the main cause.

Signs and symptoms: Most people with diverticulosis do not have any symptoms. Those who do may experience discomfort in the lower abdomen, bloating, constipation, and cramps. Diverticulitis is characterized by abdominal pain, tenderness in the lower left side of the abdomen (usually severe and comes on suddenly, but it can be mild and grow worse over days), cramping, nausea, vomiting, fever, chills, and change in bowel habits.

DOWN SYNDROME
Tests that help diagnose or screen for this condition: amniocentesis (screening before birth); after birth, diagnosis can be confirmed using a chromosome study (karyotype), which shows the chromosomes grouped by size, number, and shape.

Down syndrome is a genetic condition in which individuals are born with 47 chromosomes instead of the normal 46. The condition causes delays in intellectual and physical development. Down syndrome occurs in approximately 1 in every 800 live births and is the most frequently occurring chromosomal disorder.

Signs and symptoms: low muscle tone, single crease across the palm of the hand, slightly flattened facial profile, upward slant to the eyes.

GALLSTONES
Tests that help diagnose or screen for this condition: complete blood count (indicated by an elevated white blood cell count, abnormal liver enzymes, and/or excess bilirubin), abdominal ultrasound; also computed tomography (CT), radionuclide scan.

Gallstones are solid deposits of calcium salts or cholesterol that develop in the gallbladder or in the nearby bile ducts. People at greatest risk of developing gallstones include those who are older, female, or overweight, or individuals who have lost a lot of weight rapidly or who eat a very low calorie diet.

Complications from gallstones can be very serious if not treated. Blockage of the common bile duct, for example, can lead to an inflamed gallbladder (cholecystitis) or an infection of the bile duct (cholangitis). Obstruction of the common bile duct near the pancreatic duct can cause blockage in the pancreatic duct or an inflamed pancreas (acute pancreatitis). Severe acute pancreatitis can be lethal. People with gallstones are also more likely to develop gallbladder cancer.

Signs and symptoms: chronic indigestion (e.g., nausea, gas, bloating, abdominal pain); upper abdominal pain (sudden, steady and moderate to severe pain in the upper middle or upper right abdomen may signal a gallbladder attack); nausea and vomiting, fever. Symptoms of gallstones in the bile duct include pain, yellowing of the skin and white of the eyes (jaundice), clay-colored stool, fever.

GLAUCOMA
Tests that help diagnose or screen for this condition: tonometry.

Glaucoma is a group of eye diseases that can result in a loss of vision and blindness. It occurs when too much fluid pressure builds up inside the eye and damages the optic nerve, which is responsible for transmitting images to the brain. If the pressure is not relieved, glaucoma will cause loss of vision.

There are two main types of glaucoma. Open-angle glaucoma is the most common type. In this type, the structures of the eye appear normal, but fluid does not flow properly out of the eye. Angle-closure glaucoma is less common, but it can cause a sudden accumulation of pressure in the eye. Drainage of fluid may be poor because the drainage channel is too narrow or the pupil opens too wide, which blocks the flow of fluid.

Glaucoma most often affects people older than 45 and is more common in people who have diabetes or a family history of glaucoma.

Signs and symptoms: Most people experience few or no symptoms. The first sign is often loss of peripheral or side vision, which can go undetected until late in the disease. Other symptoms should prompt immediate medical care: seeing halos around lights, vision loss, redness in the eye, nausea or vomiting, eye pain.

HAY FEVER (ALLERGIC RHINITIS)

Tests that help diagnose or screen for this condition: allergy blood test (can be a home test); also skin prick test (best done by an allergy specialist).

Hay fever, also called allergic rhinitis, is an allergic response to airborne allergens, such as dust mites, pet dander, pollen, and mold. It is one of the most common allergic conditions, affecting about 20 percent of Americans.

Some people experience hay fever symptoms all year; others have symptoms at certain times of the year, especially spring and fall. Symptoms can be mild to severe, affecting the ability to function at daily activities. Seasonal hay fever triggers include grass pollen, tree pollen, weed pollen, and spores from molds and fungi, which can be worse during warmer months. Common year-round hay fever triggers include dander from pets, cockroaches, spores from fungi and molds, and dust mites.

Signs and symptoms: watery or itchy eyes, runny nose, nasal congestion, sneezing, cough, itchy nose, itchy roof of mouth, sinus pressure, facial pain, swollen skin under the eyes, itchy throat, decreased sense of taste or smell.

HEPATITIS C
Tests that help diagnose or screen for this condition: liver function tests; also blood tests for high levels of liver enzymes.

Hepatitis C is a liver disease in which the organ is inflamed. In most cases the inflammation is the result of exposure to the hepatitis C virus. Other causes may include excessive alcohol use, injury to the liver, lack of blood supply to the liver, poisoning, use of certain medications, and viral infections such as mononucleosis or cytomegalovirus.

The hepatitis C virus is spread through direct contact with contaminated blood products, including use of intravenous drugs and shared needles, exposure to contaminated blood by health-care workers, tattooing and body piercing needles, and blood transfusions. Most people don't experience any symptoms when they are first infected with hepatitis C, although the virus remains in the liver and causes chronic inflammation. Hepatitis C can be either acute or chronic. The acute version is a short-term condition that occurs within the first 6 months after you are exposed to the hepatitis C virus. Most people who get acute hepatitis C go on to develop chronic infection. Chronic hepatitis C can lead to more serious conditions, including cirrhosis (scarring of the liver), liver cancer, and even death.

No vaccine for hepatitis C has been developed. The best way to prevent the disease is to avoid behaviors that can spread the disease, such as injected drug use.

Signs and symptoms: Although hepatitis C usually doesn't cause symptoms during the early stages, some people do experience mild fatigue, achy joints and muscles, nausea, loss of appetite, and tenderness of the liver. Even as the disease progresses, symptoms may still not be present. When they do, they may include more pronounced fatigue, vomiting, jaundice (yellowing of the skin and eyes), and low-grade fever (up to 102°F).

HERNIATED DISC

Tests that help diagnose or screen for this condition: electromyography; also X-rays, computed tomography (CT), magnetic resonance imaging (MRI).

A herniated disc (or disk; also commonly referred to as a slipped disc or ruptured disc) is a condition in which a disc—one of the soft pads that lies between the bones in the spine—ruptures (herniates), pushing the center nucleus of the disc through the outer edge of the disc and toward the spinal canal. This places pressure on the nerves. A herniated disc is a common source of pain in the neck, lower back, arms, and legs.

A herniated disc can affect people of any age, but it occurs more often among people as they age, because the discs lose flexibility and begin to shrink, causing the spaces between the vertebrae to get smaller.

Signs and symptoms: A herniated disc in the lower back may be accompanied by sciatica (sharp, often shooting pain that runs from the buttocks down the back of the leg), weakness in one leg, tingling or numbness in one leg or buttock, loss of bladder or bowel control, burning pain in the neck. When the neck is affected, signs and symptoms may include pain that shoots down the arm, pain in the back of the head, weakness in one arm, tingling or numbness in one arm, loss of bladder or bowel control, burning pain in the neck, arm, or shoulders.

HIGH BLOOD PRESSURE (HYPERTENSION)

Tests that help diagnose or screen for this condition: blood pressure monitoring, which can be done at home using a home monitor, or in a doctor's office, clinic, or other health facility.

According to the American Heart Association, about one-third of adults in the United States have high blood pressure, and nearly one-third of them don't even know it. High blood pressure is defined as a reading of 140/90 mmHg or higher. The higher (systolic) number represents the pressure when the heart is beating; the lower (diastolic) number represents the pressure when the heart is resting between beats. A normal, healthy blood pressure is less than 120/80 mmHg for an adult. A reading of 120–139/80–89 mmHg is considered prehypertension.

In 90–95 percent of cases of high blood pressure, the cause is not known. This type of high blood pressure is called essential hypertension. In the remaining 5–10 percent of cases, which are called secondary hypertension, the cause may be a structural abnormality of the aorta, narrowing of certain arteries, or a kidney abnormality. Uncontrolled high blood pressure can lead to heart attack, heart failure, kidney failure, or stroke.

Signs and symptoms: Hypertension is known as the "silent killer" because it typically does not cause symptoms. Although a few people who have early-stage hypertension may experience dizzy spells, nosebleeds, and dull headaches, these signs and symptoms usually don't occur until high blood pressure reaches an advanced stage.

HIGH CHOLESTEROL (HYPERCHOLESTEROLEMIA)

Tests that help diagnose or screen for this condition: lipid panel.

Hypercholesterolemia (high cholesterol) is a condition defined by a cholesterol level that is 240 mg/dL or greater. A normal cholesterol level is defined as 200 mg/dL or lower; 201–239 mg/dL is borderline high. People who have high cholesterol or who are developing high cholesterol have fatty deposits in their blood vessels.

High cholesterol can affect people of any age. According to the American Heart Association, 20 percent of adults have cholesterol levels higher than 200 mg/dL, and about 38 million more have levels greater than 240 mg/dL. More women over age 45 have high cholesterol than men. High cholesterol is becoming an increasingly greater problem among young people, including children.

Signs and symptoms: There are no symptoms of high blood pressure. However, high cholesterol can cause atherosclerosis, a potentially deadly accumulation of cholesterol and other deposits, called plaque, on the artery walls. If the arteries that supply the heart are affected, chest pain (angina) and other symptoms of coronary artery disease may result. If plaques rupture, a blood clot may form and block the flow of blood. If blood flow to the heart stops, the result is a heart attack. Stoppage of blood to the brain results in a stroke.

HIV
Tests that help diagnose or screen for this condition: HIV blood test, which can be done either using a home test kit or at health-care facilities.

Human immunodeficiency virus (HIV) is the virus that causes AIDS, or acquired immune deficiency syndrome. HIV attacks the immune system and destroys the type of white blood cells (T cells or CD4 cells) that are necessary to fight disease. As a result, people with HIV have a compromised immune system, which places them at high risk of infection.

The Centers for Disease Control and Prevention (CDC) estimates there are 1 million people in the United States living with HIV or AIDS, and that about 25 percent of them don't know they have the disease. This places them at great risk as well as those with whom they have sexual contact or share needles or other items related to their drug use if they are intravenous drug or steroid users.

Signs and symptoms: Many people who are infected with HIV do not experience any symptoms for 10 years or longer. Warning signs and symptoms of advanced HIV infection include rapid weight loss, dry cough, extreme fatigue, swollen lymph glands in the groin, neck, or armpits, diarrhea that lasts for more than seven days, pneumonia, memory loss, depression, recurring fever or severe night sweats, white spots or unusual blemishes in the mouth or throat, and red, brown, pink, or purple spots on or under the skin or inside the nose, mouth, or eyelids.

HYPERTHYROIDISM
Tests that help diagnose or screen for this condition: thyroid panel, thyroid nuclear medicine tests.

Testing is especially important for older adults, who often do not have classic symptoms of the disease.

Hyperthyroidism is a condition in which the thyroid gland is overactive, producing too much of the hormone thyroxine. This can occur for several reasons, including:

- Graves disease, an autoimmune disorder in which antibodies produced by the immune system prompt the thyroid to produce an excessive amount of thyroxine. This is the most common cause of hyperthyroidism.

- Hyperfunctioning thyroid nodules, which occurs when one or more adenomas (a benign lump) of the thyroid produce too much thyroxine.

- Thyroiditis, in which the thyroid gland becomes inflamed for reasons unknown. The inflammation can cause excess thyroid hormone to leak into the bloodstream.

Hyperthyroidism can lead to complications, including heart problems (e.g., rapid heart rate), brittle bones (osteoporosis), eye problems, swollen skin, and thyrotoxic crisis (sudden intensification of symptoms that leads to fever, rapid pulse, and sometimes delirium).

Signs and symptoms: Weight loss, rapid heart rate, nervousness, diarrhea, sensitivity to heat, changes in bowel patterns (especially more frequent bowel movements), irregular menstrual periods, fatigue, muscle weakness, sleep problems. An uncommon problem called Graves ophthalmopathy may affect the eyes. In this disorder, the eyeballs protrude, and the eyes may be red and swollen. Other symptoms include blurry or double vision, sensitivity to light, and excessive tearing.

HYPOTHYROIDISM
Tests that help diagnose or screen for this condition: thyroid panel, thyroid nuclear medicine tests.

Hypothyroidism is a condition in which the thyroid gland, which is located in the neck, produces an inadequate amount of thyroid hormones. People of any age can get hypothyroidism, but it is more common among older adults. Women age 60 and older have the highest risk.

Hypothyroidism may be caused by a number of different factors, including:

• Autoimmune disease (Hashimoto's thyroiditis), when the immune system produces antibodies that attack the thyroid. This is the most common cause of hypothyroidism. Why this autoimmune response occurs is not known.

- Radiation therapy used to treat cancers of the neck and head can impact the thyroid and cause hypothyroidism.

- Treatment for hyperthyroidism, including radioactive iodine or antithyroid drugs, can result in permanent hypothyroidism.

- Thyroid surgery can reduce or eliminate hormone production and require you to take thyroid hormones for life.

- Medications, such as lithium, can affect the thyroid gland function.

If hypothyroidism is not treated, it can lead to a number of problems, including goiter (enlarged thyroid gland), heart problems, depression, slowed mental functioning, infertility, and birth defects.

Signs and symptoms: Weight gain, tiredness, feeling of being too cold, frequent menstrual periods, dry skin, brittle nails, constipation, weakness. Left untreated, hypothyroidism can raise cholesterol levels and increase the risk of a heart attack or stroke.

INFLAMMATORY BOWEL DISEASE
Tests that help diagnose or screen for this condition: fecal occult test, complete blood count, barium enema, colonoscopy.

Inflammatory bowel disease is a term that covers a group of disorders in which the intestines are inflamed. The two main types of IBD are ulcerative colitis and Crohn's disease. Ulcerative colitis affects the colon (large intestine) while Crohn's disease can involve any part of the gastrointestinal tract from the mouth to the anus, although it usually impacts the small intestine and/or the colon.

It is estimated that 1–2 million people in the United States have some kind of inflammatory bowel disease. There are several theories about the causes of inflammatory bowel disease, but an exact cause is still unknown. One popular theory is that bacteria in the intestinal tract interact with the immune system and trigger an inflammatory response. Although cigarette smoking is a known risk factor for Crohn's disease, it is protective in ulcerative colitis. Scientists have found that certain genetic mutations make people more likely to develop inflammatory bowel disease, but these mutations alone are not enough to cause the disease. The disease is more common among Caucasians and Jews than African Americans, Asians, Hispanics, or Native Americans.

Signs and symptoms: Can range from mild to severe and may include abdominal cramps and pain, bloody diarrhea, severe urgency to have a bowel movement, fever, loss of appetite, weight loss, anemia (from blood loss). Intestinal complications may include profuse bleeding from the ulcers, rupture of the bowel, strictures and/or fistulae (more common in Crohn's disease).

LUNG CANCER

Tests that help diagnose or screen for this condition: bronchoscopy; also chest X-rays, sputum analysis, computed tomography, magnetic resonance imaging.

Lung cancer is the presence of uncontrolled growth of abnormal cells in one or both lungs. The abnormal cells can form tumors and hinder the function of the lung.

There are two main types of lung cancer: nonsmall cell and small cell lung cancer. Non-small cell lung cancer (NSCLC) accounts for about 80 percent of all lung cancer cases. The different types of NSCLC include squamous cell carcinoma (the most common type of NSCLC); adenocarcinoma, and large-cell undifferentiated carcinoma. The other main type of lung cancer, small-cell lung cancer, accounts for about 20 percent of all lung cancers. It can spread quickly and form large tumors throughout the body.

Lung cancer is one of the most common cancers. In 2007, the disease accounted for approximately 15 percent of all cancer diagnoses and 29 percent of all cancer deaths. It is the number one cause of death from cancer in both men and women, with the disease affecting more men than women. The average age of people who receive a diagnosis of lung cancer is 69 years.

Signs and symptoms: These can take years to develop and may not appear until the disease is in advanced stages. Some symptoms that can occur in the chest include coughing, especially if persistent or intense; pain in the chest, shoulder, or back unrelated to pain from coughing; change in volume or color of sputum; shortness of breath; hoarseness or changes in the voice; recurrent lung problems such as bronchitis; coughing up phlegm or mucus, especially with blood; harsh sounds with each breath. Symptoms that may occur elsewhere in the body include loss of appetite, unexplained weight loss, fatigue, unsteady gait, neck or facial swelling, general weakness, blood clots, headache, bone or joint pain.

MUSCULAR DYSTROPHY

Tests that help diagnose or screen for this condition: electromyography, complete blood count; also ultrasonography, muscle biopsy.

Muscular dystrophy is a general term for a group of more than 30 genetic diseases characterized by progressive weakness and degeneration of muscles that control movement. The various disorders differ in terms of the severity and location of the muscle weakness, age of onset, how fast the disease progresses, and the pattern of inheritance. Some of the more common types include:

- Duchenne: The most common form, it usually first appears between ages 3 and 5 years and progresses rapidly. It primarily affects boys. About 20–30 boys of every 100,000 born are affected by Duchenne muscular dystrophy.

• Facioscapulohumeral: Usually begins in adolescence and progresses slowly. Weakness occurs in the face, arms, legs, and around the shoulders and chest.

• Myotonic: The most common adult form, characterized by prolonged muscle spasms, cataracts, cardiac abnormalities, and endocrine problems.

Signs and symptoms: These vary depending on the type of muscular dystrophy. Generally, symptoms may include muscle weakness, lack of coordination, and progressive crippling that results in loss of mobility. Specific signs and symptoms for the three more common forms are provided here:

• **Duchenne:** frequent falls, large calf muscles, difficulty rising from a lying or sitting position, waddling gait, mild mental retardation (in some cases), weak lower leg muscles.

• **Facioscapulohumeral:** progressive muscle weakness, usually in this order: face, shoulders, abdomen, feet, upper arms, pelvis, lower arms.

- **Myotonic:** inability to relax muscles at will (myotonia), weakening of voluntary muscles that control arms, legs, head, neck, face, breathing, and swallowing; fainting or dizziness; weakening of muscles of hollow internal organs (e.g., uterus, stomach); difficulty sleeping; daytime sleepiness; cataracts; mild diabetes.

OSTEOPOROSIS

Tests that help diagnose or screen for this condition: The best screening test for osteoporosis is a dual-energy X-ray absorptiometry (DEXA) scan. It is quick, accurate, and easy to use. The peripheral test, which scans the heel, is less accurate.

Osteoporosis is a condition in which the bones become weak and brittle, placing them at high risk of fracturing. Most of the fractures occur in the spine, hip, or wrist. Osteoporosis is usually the result of low levels of calcium, phosphorus, magnesium, and other minerals in your bones.

Although it is commonly thought of as a woman's disease, it affects men as well. Osteoporosis is a major public health threat for an estimated 44 million Americans (55% of people 50 years and older). Approximately 10 million Americans already have the disease (approximately 80% are women), and nearly 34 million more are believed to have low bone mass, which places them at increased risk for osteoporosis.

Signs and symptoms: Often none until a fracture occurs. Some people experience back pain.

PROSTATE CANCER

Tests that help diagnose or screen for this condition: prostate-specific antigen (PSA) test; also digital rectal examination, cystoscopy, prostate ultrasound.

Prostate cancer is cancer that forms in the tissues of the prostate gland, which is found below the bladder and in front of the rectum in males. It is the most common type of cancer in males. According to the National Cancer Institute, an estimated 186,320 new cases of prostate cancer occurred in the United States in 2008. This form of cancer usually occurs in men older than 50.

The causes of prostate cancer are unknown. The hormone testosterone does not cause the disease and is believed to have little or no role in tumor growth. Scientists are investigating the possibility that certain genes may play a role, and a diet high in saturated fat has been suggested to play a part as well.

Signs and symptoms: Early prostate cancer has no warning signs or symptoms. Once a malignant tumor forms, it can cause the prostate gland to become enlarged. Symptoms of blockage as a result of the cancer growth include frequent need to urinate, difficulty starting or stopping urination, weak or interrupted urination, painful or burning sensation during urination or ejaculation, blood in urine or semen. Symptoms of advanced prostate cancer include dull, incessant deep pain or stiffness in the pelvic region, lower back, ribs, or upper thighs; weight loss; loss of appetite; fatigue; nausea and/or vomiting.

PSORIASIS
Tests that help diagnose or screen for this condition: skin biopsy.

Psoriasis is a chronic, noncontagious autoimmune disease in which there is a malfunction in the growth cycle of skin cells. The result is an excessive buildup of abnormal skin in various parts of the body. The National Institutes of Health reports that as many as 7.5 million Americans have psoriasis in one of its five forms: plaque, guttate, inverse, pustular, and erythrodermic. Plaque psoriasis is the most common, affecting about 80 percent of people who have the disease.

The cause of psoriasis is related to the activity of a type of white blood cell called T lymphocyte, or T cell. Normally, T cells detect and destroy foreign elements, such as bacteria or viruses. In psoriasis, T cells attack healthy skin cells. These overactive T cells can trigger other responses, such as dilating blood vessels around the plaques and increasing the number of white blood cells that enter the skin. Currently experts do not know what causes T cells to malfunction, although they suspect environmental and genetic factors are both involved.

Signs and symptoms:

- **Plaque psoriasis:** Raised, inflamed red lesions covered by a white silvery scale, typically found on the knees, elbows, scalp, and lower back.

- **Guttate psoriasis:** Small, red individual spots usually on the limbs and trunk. They are not usually as thick as plaque lesions.

- **Inverse psoriasis:** Very red, often smooth and shiny lesions that do not have the scale associated with plaque psoriasis. Found in the groin, armpits, under the breasts, and in other skin folds.

- **Pustular psoriasis:** White pustules (blisters of pus) surrounded by red skin. May be localized to certain areas of the body or generalized, covering most of the body.

- **Erythrodermic psoriasis:** Fiery redness and shedding of the skin that often affects most of the body. Usually accompanied by severe pain and itching.

SKIN CANCER

Tests that help diagnose or screen for this condition: skin biopsy.

According to the National Cancer Institute and the Centers for Disease Control and Prevention, skin cancer is the most common of all cancers in the United States. Most cases of skin cancer are caused by excessive exposure to the sun and appear in people who are older than 50, although skin damage caused by the sun begins at an early age. Each year in the United States, more than 1 million cases of nonmelanoma skin cancer are diagnosed. Melanoma, the most serious type of skin cancer, represents 4 percent of all skin cancer cases in the U.S., but they make up more than 75 percent of all deaths from skin cancer. Basal cell carcinoma is the most common skin cancer.

The good news is that both basal and squamous cell skin cancers have a 95 percent cure rate if they are detected and treated during their early phase.

Signs and symptoms: These depend on the type of cancer.

- **Basal cell:** Usually appears as one of the following: pearly or waxy bump on the face, neck, or ears; flat, flesh-colored or brown scarlike lesion on the back or chest.

- **Squamous cell:** Can appear as a firm, red nodule on the face, neck, ears, lips, hands, or arms; or as a flat lesion with scaly, crusted surface on the face, ears, neck, hands, or arms.

- **Melanoma:** This form can develop anywhere on the body. Warning signs include:
  large brownish spot with darker speckles;
  simple mole that changes color, size, or feel
  or that bleeds; small lesion with an irregular
  border and red, white, blue, or black spots
  on the limbs or trunk; dark lesions on the
  palms, soles, fingertips, or toes, or on the
  mucous membranes of the mouth, nose, vagina, or anus.

SPINA BIFIDA
**Tests that help diagnose or screen for this condi-
tion:** amniocentesis.

Spina bifida is the most common type of neural
tube birth defect. It begins in the womb just a few
weeks after conception, usually before women
know they are pregnant. It can occur in three
forms:

- Spina bifida occulta. In this form the defect
  is not visible, and it rarely is associated with
  symptoms or complications. It affects about
  5 percent of those with the defect.

- Meningocele: In this form the membrane
  that surrounds the spinal cord may enlarge.
  It is often not visible through the skin and
  causes no complications. It is uncommon.

• Spina bifida cystic: This is the most severe form of spina bifida and accounts for 94 percent of cases.

Spina bifida occurs in about 7 out of every 10,000 live births. The Spina Bifida Association of America estimates that there are more than 70,000 people in the United States living with the defect.

Signs and symptoms: These refer to complications for spina bifida cystic: leg paralysis, scoliosis, bowel and bladder control problems, imbalances in muscle strength, hydrocephalus, leg or foot deformities, hip dislocation, pathologic bone fractures.

URINARY TRACT INFECTION
Tests that help diagnose or screen for this condition: urinalysis; may be followed by a urine culture.

A urinary tract infection is an infection that affects the urinary system, which includes the kidneys, ureters, bladder, and urethra. Although the infection can affect the entire system, it usually involves the lower portion only—the urethra and the bladder.

Women are at greater risk of developing a urinary tract infection than men. Failure to properly treat a urinary tract infection may result in it spreading to the kidneys, which generally is a more serious condition.

Signs and symptoms: Not everyone who develops a urinary tract infection has recognizable signs and symptoms, but most people have some. These can include a persistent urge to urinate, burning sensation when urinating, passing frequent but small amounts of urine, strong-smelling urine, cloudy urine, bloody urine, bacteria in the urine. More specific signs and symptoms are associated with the type of urinary tract infection you have. Infection that affects the urethra (urethritis) is accompanied by burning when urinating. When the bladder is affected (cystitis), pelvic pressure, discomfort in the lower abdomen, low-grade fever, and frequent, painful urination are common. When the kidneys are affected (acute pyelonephritis), signs and symptoms may include high fever, shaking and chills, nausea and vomiting, and upper back and flank pain.

GLOSSARY

Bilirubin: The yellowish or orange pigment in bile. When it accumulates, it can cause jaundice.

Blood urea nitrogen: Urea nitrogen is the substance that forms when protein breaks down in the body. A test for blood levels of urea nitrogen is done to check kidney function.

Breast self-examination: An examination women age 20 and older are urged to perform by health experts to look for lumps and other breast changes. The test should be done monthly. A breast self-exam is not a substitute for regular breast examinations from a doctor or from screening mammograms.

Chemistry panel: A battery of tests that includes determining the levels of:

- fasting glucose, for evaluation of diabetes

- uric acid, for evaluation of gout or recurrent urinary stones (calculi)

- BUN (blood urea nitrogen), which directly measures liver function and indirectly assesses renal function and glomerular filtration rate

- Creatinine, which estimates glomerular filtration rate and monitors progression of renal disease

- BUN/creatinine ratio, to diagnose impaired renal function and also help monitor individuals on dialysis

- Sodium, to evaluate and monitor electrolyte and fluid balance and treatment

- Potassium, to evaluate and monitor electrolyte balance

- Chloride, which provides indication of acid-base balance and status of hydration

- Calcium, to evaluate calcium metabolism and function of the parathyroid

- Phosphorus, which measures serum phosphorus

- Protein/albumin/globulin, which helps detect diseases that affect blood proteins

- Albumin/globulin ratio, to evaluate renal disease and other chronic diseases

- Bilirubin, to evaluate liver function

- Alkaline phosphatase, to detect and monitor bone and/or liver disease

- LDH (lactic dehydrogenase), measures LDH which, when in the blood, can support detection of disease or injury

- AST (SGOT or aspartate aminotransferase), to evaluate the possibility of coronary occlusive heart disease or liver disease

- ALT (SGPT or alanine aminotransferase), to identify liver disease

- Iron, to evaluate many conditions such as iron deficiency anemia and hemochromatosis

- Cholesterol, to identify the risk of high cholesterol (hyperlipidemia) and coronary heart disease

- Triglycerides, to identify the risk of developing coronary heart disease or fat metabolism disorders

- HDL cholesterol, which measures alpha lipoprotein and helps to predict heart disease

- LDL cholesterol, which measures beta lipoprotein and helps to predict heart disease

- Total cholesterol/HDL ratio, used to determine the risk for coronary heart disease

Computed tomography: A computed tomography (CT) scan is an imaging technique that uses X-rays to produce cross-sectional pictures of the body.

Cushing's syndrome: A condition characterized by moon face, high blood pressure, emotional disturbances, weight gain, and in women, abnormal growth of body hair. It is caused by abnormally high levels of the hormone cortisol.

Cystoscopy: A procedure that allows clinicians to see inside the bladder and urethra. It is performed using a cystoscope, a specially designed endoscope (a type of tube) that has a small camera on the end.

Digital rectal exam: An examination of the lower rectum performed by a physician. The doctor uses a gloved, lubricated finger to check for lumps or other abnormalities. In females this is often done during a pelvic examination.

Echocardiogram: A test that uses sound waves to produce a real-time picture of the heart. An echocardiogram provides much greater detail than an X-ray and does not involve radiation.

Glomerulonephritis: Inflammation of the kidney accompanied by inflammation of the capillary loops in the kidney.

Glomerular filtration rate: A measurement of the amount of glomerular filtrate (a substance similar to blood plasma but without proteins) that forms in the kidneys each minute. This test is used to evaluate the ability of the kidneys to eliminate waste products from the body, to look for early signs of kidney damage, and for signs of deterioration in kidney function in people who have kidney disease.

Keratoses: Growths that develop on the skin. There are two main types: seborrheic and actinic. Seborrheic keratoses are noncancerous; they are usually brown but can range in color from tan to black. Actinic keratoses are precancerous growths and are usually caused by excessive exposure to the sun.

Magnetic resonance imaging (MRI): A noninvasive test that uses powerful magnets and radio waves to take images of the body.

Prevalence rate: The number of people in a population who have a disease or specific health condition at a given time.

Radionuclide scan: A technique used to take images of the body by using a small dose of a radioactive substance and a scanner to track where the substance goes.

Sigmoidoscopy: An internal examination of the lower large bowel (colon) that requires use of an instrument called a sigmoidoscope.

APPENDIX

RESOURCES FOR FURTHER INFORMATION
For more information about diagnostic and screening tests and the diseases and medical conditions for which they are done, please contact your healthcare provider or refer to the organizations, Web sites, and literature listed below. There is a separate list of home test kit information.

Organizations and Web Sites
American Academy of Allergy, Asthma & Immunology
http://www.aaaai.org

American Academy of Ophthalmology
http://www.aao.org

American Autoimmune Related Diseases Association
http://www.aarda.org

American Cancer Society
http://www.cancer.org

American College of Gastroenterology
http://www.acg.gi.org

American Diabetes Association
http://www.diabetes.org

American Gastroenterological Association
http://www.gastro.org

American Heart Association
http://www.americanheart.org

American Institute of Ultrasound in Medicine
http://www.aium.org

American Society for Dermatologic Surgery
http://www.asds-net.org

American Society of Radiologic Technologists
http://www.asrt.org

American Thyroid Association
http://www.thyroid.org

U.S. Food and Drug Administration
http://www.fda.gov

Lab Tests Online
http://www.labtestsonline.org

March of Dimes Foundation
http://www.marchofdimes.com

Mayo Clinic
http://www.mayoclinic.com

Muscular Dystrophy Association
http://www.mda.org

National Cancer Institute
http://www.cancer.gov/

National Heart, Lung, and Blood Institute
http://www.nhlbi.nih.gov

National Institute of Allergy and Infectious Diseases
http://www.niaid.nih.gov

National Institute of Arthritis and Musculoskeletal
and Skin Diseases
http://www.niams.nih.gov

National Institute of Neurological Disorders and
Stroke
http://www.ninds.nih.gov/

Publications

Beers, Mark H. et al. *The Merck Manual 18th Edition*. Merck, 2006.

Johnson, David, et al. *Medical Tests That Can Save Your Life: 21 Tests Your Doctor Won't Order . . . Unless You Know to Ask*. Rodale, 2004.

Margolis, Simeon. *The Johns Hopkins Consumer Guide to Medical Tests: What You Can Expect, How You Should Prepare, What Your Results Mean*. Rebus Inc., 2001.

McPhee, Stephen and Maxine Papadakis. *Current Medical Diagnosis and Treatment 2009*. (LANGE CURRENT series). McGraw-Hill, 2008.

Pasricha P. J. "Gastrointestinal endoscopy." In: Goldman L., Ausiello D., et. al., eds. *Cecil Medicine 23rd ed*. Philadelphia: Saunders Elsevier, 2008; chapter 136.

Segen, Joseph C. and Josie Wade Owens. *The Patient's Guide to Medical Tests: Everything You Need to Know About the Tests Your Doctor Orders*. Facts on File, 2002.

ONLINE SOURCES OF HOME TEST KITS

Here are a few online sources of home test kits. You can also find home test kits at your local pharmacy and in some health food stores.

All Test Kits
http://www.alltestkits.com/
Providers of allergy, cholesterol, diabetes, illegal drugs, kidney, thyroid, and other home test kits.

Drug Testing World
http://www.drugtestingworld.com/
Suppliers of urine, saliva, and hair drug testing kits, from single to 12-panel kits; also pregnancy and ovulation test kits.

HealthGoods, LLC
http://www.healthgoods.com/shopping/home_test_kits/Home_Test_Kits.htm
Allergy test kit, lead test kit, among others.

Home Drug Testing Kit
http://www.homedrugtestingkit.com/
Provides FDA-approved home testing kits for alcohol and drugs.

Home Health Testing
http://www.homehealthtesting.com/
Suppliers of drug, tobacco, and alcohol test kits.

Test Country
http://www.testcountry.com/
Provider of all the home test kits discussed in this book.

Test Medical Symptoms @ Home, Inc.
http://www.testsymptomsathome.com/

Supplier of home devices, instant tests, and laboratory tests.

USA Drug Screening
http://www.usadrugscreening.com/
Online suppliers of urine and saliva drug test kits.

Virginia Hopkins Health Watch Test Kits
http://www.virginiahopkinstestkits.com/testsleadin
.html
Carries test kits for vitamin D, colorectal cancer, hormone levels, and more.

ZRT Laboratory
http://www.zrtlab.com/
Carries test kits for hormone levels, Vitamin D, and more.